THE *NEW* MIRACLES
OF REBOUND EXERCISE

THE *NEW* MIRACLES
OF REBOUND EXERCISE

Albert Earl Carter

A.L.M. Publishers
Scottsdale, Arizona 85260

THE *NEW* MIRACLES OF REBOUND EXERCISE

ISBN: 0-9619041-2-7

Printed in the United States of America

Disclaimer

This book is informational only and should not be considered a substitute for consultation with a duly licensed medical doctor. Any attempt to diagnose and treat an illness should come under the direction of a physician. The author is not a medical doctor and does not purport to offer medical advise, make diagnoses, prescribe remedies for specific medical conditions, or substitute for medical consultation.

TABLE OF CONTENTS

INTRODUCTION

"It looks too simple to be any good."

That is probably the biggest argument against it. How could anything so simple be so good for you? If rebound exercise was a little more complicated or caused greater discomfort, like other accepted modes of exercise, it would probably be more popular because we have come to expect that from our exercises. But it is simple, and it doesn't cause pain. The fact is, it just happens to be the most effective way to efficiently tap three major forces simultaneously. . . forces that have not previously been considered when we exercise.

We invite you to become one of the thousands who, each month, are discovering this unique method of eliminating bone-jarring, sometimes crippling shock, to their weight-bearing joints and still achieving their aerobic requirements. As you consider rebounding, you will begin to understand how some of our best athletes are using rebounding to hone their individual athletic skills. But, unlike many other exercise methods, rebounding is not just for the athlete. Rather, it is universal in scope; from the pregnant lady, to the muscle-bound athlete, to the overweight, out-of-shape executive.

1

We also include a word on therapeutic rebounding, because we have found rebound exercise to be an excellent tool for those who are not able to exercise in conventional, or accepted ways.

It was not too long ago, say mid '70s, if you saw somebody running in the middle of a busy city, it was because the police were after him. In fact, it was just before Dr. Kenneth Cooper introduced us to the word 'aerobics'. That was the beginning of the exercise explosion. Accountants, bankers, doctors, and other blue and white collar workers could now calculate 'aerobic points'. Nike of Beaverton, Oregon invented the 'spikeless running shoe' and America was off to the races. Marathons and ten-K's here we come! We have been running ever since, although there is good evidence showing that running is not what it was supposed to be - a utopian exercise.

This book is not being written to run down running, weight lifting, aerobic dance, calisthenics, or any other form of exercise. We choose not to run down other activities simply because it is not necessary. If your type of exercise is injurious, ineffective, or inconvenient you'll find out soon enough. When you do, you'll be looking around for something to take its place because, most of the time, people are healthier, happier and feel better about themselves and the rest of their world when they are involved with a good exercise program.

At the very least, you will find that rebounding is an excellent adjunct to your already ongoing exercise program. At its best, you will find that rebounding goes beyond your wildest expectations, making all other exercise methods obsolete. You read right. Rebounding is by far the most efficient, the most effective form of exercise yet devised by man. That statement was made in 1977, when we published the small book, *Rebound to Better Health*. Since then, that statement has been challenged by some of the best scientists in the world, and endorsed by some of the best athletes. The results are always the same. When the learned take the time to understand the full implications of rebound exercise, they say, "Yup, you are right."

Most revolutionary concepts are usually simple. The lasting ones are true. However, our advanced scientific ego demands that all new ideas must be conceived in a laboratory test tube after years of investigative research. The new idea must then be incubated by sophisticated engineers of industry until rendered completely safe and harmless, ready for public consumption. It is then mass-marketed by some conglomerate.

We consumers accept this as part of life, so much so that, until a simple truth stands up in front of us and slaps us in the face, it seldom gets our attention. But, when it does, we murmur to ourselves, "Gee. That is so true. . . and so simple! I wish I'd thought of that!" Rebound exercise is one of those simple, logical truths that belong to all of us. Only this time, we said something about it.

The first publication of *The Miracles of Rebound Exercise* rolled off the press near the end of 1979, after over a dozen publishing companies turned the manuscript down, saying that it wouldn't sell because the only people who would buy the book would be those who owned one of those 'springy things'. So it became necessary for us to publish it ourselves.

We were in Australia, near the end of 1981, to lecture about the benefits of rebounding. A major complaint from the Aussies was that they had to wait six weeks to get the book shipped from the United States. A simple solution was to have it printed 'down under'. A phone call to a publishing company went something like this:

"Hi, this is Mr. Carter, from the U.S. We would like to have you print my book here in Australia."

"Oh, what is your book about?"

"Exercise."

"There's a lot of people writing about that now, isn't there?"

"I suppose so, but mine is different."

"I know, that's what they all say. How many copies have you sold?"

"One million three hundred thousand."

"That's great! You must have a good publisher. Who publishes your book in the states?"

"We do."

"Then, you must have a great distributing company. Who distributes it for you?"

"We do."

"Man! You must have an excellent advertising campaign. Who does your advertising?"

"We do, but I don't have an advertising budget."

"Then, you must have a great book. Why don't you come in this afternoon?"

At its very best, the original *Miracles,* was an amateur effort - written, published, and distributed by amateurs. The book was successful in spite of all odds because of the truth of the message. The message in this book is the same, only this time we have ten years of proof that we have a valid concept. A medical doctor in Australia exclaimed, "This could be the greatest medical breakthrough of this decade!" Time will tell.

Albert E. Carter

CHAPTER 1

TESTIMONIALS

I have to smile. . . no. . . chuckle as I begin to write about some of the testimonials about rebound exercise. I remember in '78 rebounding was so young, I had to search all over the known world for people who had a positive experience because of rebounding. I included the testimonials as the last chapter of the original *Miracles* for two reasons: it gave me more time to accumulate the personal experiences while I wrote the rest of the book; and it was a final way to say to the unbelievers, "I'm not the only strange one."

A strange thing happened. As some of my readers loaned my book to their friends, they would tell my prospective readers, "Read the last chapter first." So, simple deduction convinced me that what the readers want to read first should be at the front of the book.

Let's see. Where should we begin? Unlike '78, there's so many. We could start at the top:

When President Ronald Reagan was asked how he kept in shape, he answered, "When I'm out at the ranch, I cut down trees. But here in Washington, they frown on Presidents who cut down trees. I find it necessary to exercise indoors for security reasons. I have a little rebounder I use to get my exercise. So, if you see somebody jumping up and down on the second floor of the White House, that's me rebounding."

Now, I know that's not going to cut it for at least fifty percent of the voting population at any one time, so how about somebody we all love? "I keep my rebounder at the foot of my bed and use it daily." - *Bob Hope..*

How about a medical endorsement: "Never in my 35 years as a practicing physician have I found any exercise method, for any price, that will do more for the physical body than rebound exercise." - *Henry Savage, M.D.*

Another writer of contemporary literature: "Rebound exercise is the closest thing to the Fountain of Youth that science has found." *James R. White,* PhD, author of *Jump for Joy,* 1981.

Maybe you would prefer to hear from some of the scientists who challenged the concept of rebound exercise. "The external work output at equivalent levels of oxygen uptake were significantly greater while trampolining than running . . . the greatest difference was about 68%" — *NASA* - Ames Research Center, Moffett Field, California, study published in the *Journal of Applied Physiology* 49(5):881-887, 1980.

Of course, you can always find someone with a reputation who will endorse an idea if the price is right. Maybe you would like to hear from people who are classified as just good people.

Actually, I could go on and on with real live drama about the rebound. In fact, I have been threatening to write a book that would include only real happenings to real people with real rebounders. Maybe I will, after I have written the ones I have been commissioned to write.

The LaVern Groff Story

" 'And they were married and lived happily ever after.' Some fairy tales end that way, but the first seven years of my married life were a nightmare. I was in and out of hospitals more times than I could remember. Less than a year after we were married, my ovary had ruptured and I was bleeding internally. The removal of half the ovary was followed a year later by another operation which removed the other half. Some things come in threes. It was less than a year later and I was back in the hospital for my third operation. This time I lost half of the other ovary. In the recovery room, my heart stopped. The quick action of the staff started it beating again.

"After everything my body went through, I guess I don't blame it for just giving up. My nerves and muscles no longer functioned. I became a vegetable for over two months. Someone had to feed me because I didn't have strength to even lift my arms, and walking was impossible. My back muscles were so weak that I was in constant pain. As I began to learn how to walk all over again, I desperately prayed, 'Oh, Lord. Isn't there any hope for me?'

"The Lord does answer prayers. Shortly thereafter, my husband and I were introduced to rebound exercise while attending a self-help clinic. Dr. Corwin West gave us therapeutic instructions and we took a rebounder home with us.

"At first, I had to sit on the rebounder with my husband standing behind me providing the bounce. In a few weeks, I found I could sit and rebound myself by moving my arms. Soon I could stand and gently bounce. As the months went by, I could feel the strength coming back. It was almost like climbing out of a dark grave into a meadow of flowers. I was glad to be alive! Not only were my arms and legs getting stronger, I could actually feel my insides getting stronger. My pain was disappearing. After using the rebounder for a year, we wouldn't give it up for all the world. I want everyone to know this is the best thing for eliminating pain without pills. I am now rebounding up to 15 minutes several times a day and feel just wonderful."

NOTE: LaVerne Groff gave birth to a six-pound baby a few

months after writing her story for us. Because of her previous health problems, her doctors were on the lookout for complications, but they found the baby to be perfectly healthy. Needless to say, Dad is just as proud as a peacock!

The Walt and Dorothy Ross Story

"My name is Dorothy Ross and I'm not going to tell you how old I am, but I am a proud grandmother of 21 beautiful grandbabies. . . and I feel as good right now as I did when I was 35, but that wasn't true for the last few hard years before.

"When I was hospitalized for a pinched nerve, my arthritis spread to my right knee and both ankles. I had bursitis in the right shoulder and both hips. I began to suffer with constant back aches and always felt completely exhausted. Other problems plagued me, too, and the years seemed long with headaches, high-blood pressure, ringing in my ears and poor balance.

"Mind you, all this had been going on for years on end. I was contantly under a doctor's care. He told me I was just getting old and had to expect this sort of thing.

"Walt had severe and painful problems, too. He suffered a heart attack, was found to be a diabetic and had four cancer surgeries last year.

"I worried about Walt and he worried about me. We were just sick and tired about being sick and tired.

"After a week of fervent prayer, Walt brought home a rebounder. He was excited, but I was skeptical. For three days I watched him bounce for thirty seconds at a time. Each day he seemed brighter and had more energy. His disposition turned happy and sunny and literally began to whistle while he worked, something I hadn't heard for a long time.

"Following his example, I tried to use the rebounder but couldn't keep my balance. Walt held my hands to steady me morning and evening for three days. Sure enough, I began to feel better too! In two weeks my blood pressure dropped

30 points! I had more stamina, and I lost 8 pounds. I began to sing while I worked - literally sing! Life took on a whole new outlook. I had hurt and been tired for so long, I had actually forgotten how it felt to feel really good - no, really great!

"After just two and a half months, my back aches and headaches were gone. No more arthritis or bursitis pain. The leg and foot cramps that woke me up every night disappeared. I went from a size 24 to a size 18!

"And listen to what rebounding has done for Walt! His stamina and recuperative powers have reached phenomenal dimensions. He lost 18 pounds. His cholesterol level is 10 points below normal. His heart rate dropped 8 beats per minute. His eyesight has cleared. He watches television and drives without glasses. The doctor says that he is now in better physical condition than any time since he has known him!

"Are we thrilled to share the unbelievable benefits of the rebounder? You bet! Our whole life has changed for the better. We are happier, healthier, busier and more eager for each new day."

The Harris Nelson Story

Harris Nelson, of Hollywood, California, former president of Hollywood's famous Comedy Club, 70 years young, sums up the benefits of rebounding in inimitable style.

"All you have to do is bounce on the rebounder, very easily at first (convalescents can sit on it), and it is astounding how it massages every organ in your body. The results are fantastic!

"The concept is new. Bouncing puts all of the cells in the body under stress. In defense, they fortify themselves by strengthening their walls. They become stronger and so do you! It's as simple as that! And it works!

"I need only six hours of sleep at night now - and no tossing as before - I wake up refreshed. No more getting up nights. Stress and anxiety reduced 100%. Cough gone. Arthritis gone.

"I can eat anything now, even before going to bed and I

don't wake up dizzy and nauseated at four in the morning because of my heart problems. NO ANGINA PAINS!

"I have never enjoyed better regularity or elimination.

"I have renewed zip and vitality.

"I've lost 8 pounds and no dieting. All muscles are firmer. My pot belly is reduced 1½ inches.

"I can read music faster. My mind reacts much quicker, and I'm sure it is correcting disorders I'm not even aware of. Plus, plus, plus!

"All this and why? Better circulation. Stronger lung power and a stimulated lymphatic system (your toxic poison and waste removal system). Action and movement. Exercise! And happy day, I can do it while watching television. No special garb, no sweat!

"And it's done all this for me in less than four months, rebounding just five minutes twice a day. That's all I need to keep fit!"

Pat Glaspie

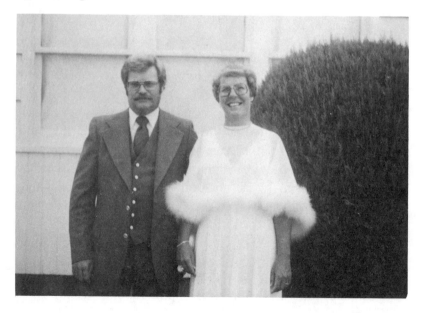

My name is Pat Glaspie and I reside in Ritzville, Washington. I was born with cerebral palsy which affected my right side. Two years ago, I was introduced to rebound exercise. After eleven days on a rebounder, I was able to wiggle two of my right toes. I was so thrilled I became very dedicated to exercising on the rebounder very faithfully. My health wasn't at all good at that time plus the fact that I was thirty pounds overweight.

Within two months, I lost 27 pounds and went from a size 16 to a size 10, and in three month's time, I was able to control my entire right foot. I now have control over my complete

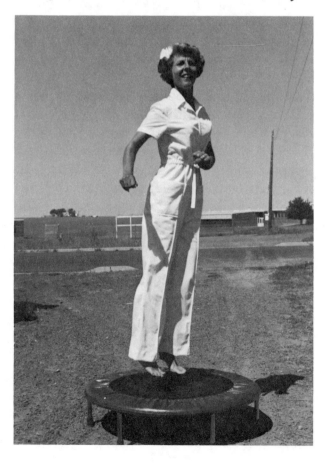

right side!

As if cerebral palsy was not affliction enough, I also had hypoglycemia and spent at least seven days each month in bed from pure exhaustion because this disease caused my heart to beat as high as 200 beats per minute. This also put me in a very despondent mood most of the time, and at times I was sure I would die before the day was over. Through much study of rebound exercise, I knew the rebounder would help this problem also.

About this same time, I attended lectures given by Dr. C. Samuel West, D.N., to learn how to eliminate poisons from the body. Between rebound exercise and Dr. West, the hypoglycemia was completely gone from my body within seven months.

I became so sold on rebounders that I had to let the rest of the world know my new-found exercise, so I began lecturing to small groups and selling rebounders.

I now lecture all over the eastern part of Washington. I like to think I am a combination of Al Carter and Dr. West. I teach diet, lymphatics and rebound exercise and today I thank the Lord that I am a new woman with a bright future of good health and financial success! What more could anyone ask?"

Enough of the testimonials for now. Let's find out about rebounding. Why is it that we have been able to accumulate these true life experiences from people of all walks of life?

CHAPTER 2

BASIC CONCEPTS OF EXERCISE

A former president of a university was quoted as saying, "When I feel the urge to exercise, I lie down until the crisis passes." Obviously the value of daily, consistent exercise has escaped the minds of a great many people. But then, there are many who swear by exercise but who still don't really understand what it is or how it can be beneficial to us. How many times have you heard, "If it doesn't hurt, it doesn't work" or, "You've got to pain and strain to gain."

The latest one to come along with the advent of TV's 20 — minute workout: "You need to exercise hard enough to keep your sustained heart rate at 80% of the maximum for 20 minutes, or it doesn't do you any good."

When asked why the Nike running shoe people endorse the "Target Zone" concept, they answered, "Because it sells running shoes and exercise clothes."

"You must work hard, sweat hard and get sore," exhorted Jane Fonda in her *Workout* in 1981. These sayings are the result of our need to follow an expert. Sadly, once we find a person who claims to be an expert, many people follow blindly without any investigation or application of common sense. For example, "If it doesn't hurt, it doesn't work." This saying is found in almost every football locker room. It was put up by the present or former coach. All high school, college and professional football players accept this saying as gospel. They don't even stop to consider that maybe that saying is for the self-gratification of the coach. You see, he has the responsibility of producing a winning football team regardless of how many students injure themselves by over-extending themselves in the process of making the first cut. Besides, young, resilient students will heal and bounce back. That is, if they want to play football, the man's sport. The real harm is not in the injury to the few students, because the coach is right. Most will heal and play. The real harm is that we now have an entire new industry, the exercise industry who's leaders were taught to pay homage to these sacred cows. After all, they learned these sayings from their coaches. Now that they are coaches themselves, they are going to emulate their coaches.

Strength — A Reason to Exercise

Most of the people who become involved in weight lifting have the desire, for whatever reason, to become stronger. They have been told of only one way. They have to be willing to pay the price. Part of that price is pain. Why? Our accepted experts will tell you "There's no other way." When a person talks of strength exercises, you can count on several underlining points. How do you challenge a specific group of voluntary muscles? What kind of movement, how many repetitions, and how many sets of repetitions are necessary to maximize the muscle-building effects on each specific group of muscles? Whether it is weight lifting with free weights, using multiple station arrangements, or the more sophisticated continuous tension through a full range of motion systems, the objective is to challenge the muscle so much that the weaker muscle cells die thus making more room for the stronger muscles cells to take their place.

The Good, the Bad, and the Ugly.

The good side of this form of exercise is that most people do not exercise hard enough to destroy the weaker muscle cells simply because it is painful. Most people don't like pain, so they experience the healthful benefits to be expected of moderate exercise programs.

The bad side is that the instructors feel that if you are not in pain the next day, you are less than the person you could be.

The ugly is that our heroes in the demanding sports of football and body building do put up with the pain of maximum body building in their effort to be a better athlete or a better human specimen. The internal destruction at the cell level is immeasurable. The bulky body is not always pure muscle. Many times, a large portion of the bulk we think of a healthy muscle is scar tissue due to the continuous damage caused by going beyond the rupture threshold of healthy cell tissues. It begins to show up when a weight trainer slows down. The average life expectancy of a professional football player is 54 years. Caution: Exercise may be hazardous to your health.

Aerobics - Another Reason to Exercise

I am convinced that Doctor Kenneth Cooper had no idea what was going to happen to the American public when he finished his first book entitled, *Aerobics,* published in 1968. Naturally, being a medical doctor, he had the credibility other doctors needed to recommend its reading to their patients. In his book, he explains that all popular exercises have been scientifically measured for the amount of energy it takes to perform them. These amounts were translated into points, and the number of points necessary to produce an optimum level of fitness was firmly established by their evaluations. Their method of evaluation? Simply measure the consumption of oxygen. In the simplest of terms, any activity requires energy. Energy is produced by burning foodstuffs. The burning, or oxidation, requires oxygen. Since the body cannot store oxygen the way it is able to store foodstuffs, the measurement of oxygen consumption is the most effective way of measuring energy production. This is why he used the term, *Aerobics* as the title of his book. It is important to note that he didn't say that certain exercises were aerobic and others were not. He simply stated that some demanded more energy utilization. Even winking demands energy and therefore, is an aerobic exercise. But the terms, 'aerobic exercise' and 'aerobic points' had a medical ring to them. They were something that could be measured. Soon, everyone who was the least bit interested in exercise, sports, or physical fitness was comparing their pet activity with others at social parties and company picnics. Chiropractors and medical doctors alike were making the book available through their offices. The marketers could not pass up this golden opportunity.

The Mass Marketers Dream

It started with the shoe manufacturers. Running shoes without spikes with special heels and soles for running on blacktop and concrete were unheard of before Cooper's *Aerobics*. The clothing manufacturers followed with their multi-colored, multi-styled, color-coordinated sweat suits. Now, all they needed was more people to get involved with 'aerobics', so the major merchandisers began to sponsor running events such as 10 K's, and marathons. The news media picked up on the herds of people who had never run before, now practicing for the run of their lives. Non-profit fund raising strategies made it almost unAmerican to say anything against it, so the foot doctors and chiropractors didn't. After all, when a runner needed medical help, where could they turn? Medical business is always good after an open-to-the-public marathon.

On July 20, 1984, James Fuller Fixx went out alone for

a ten mile run along the back roads of Vermont. At 5:30 p.m., a passing motorcyclist found the best selling author and proselytizer of fitness by running stretched atop the tarmac, dead at 52.

In 1979, the President of the United States, Jimmy Carter, suffered heart exhaustion while attempting a ten-kilometer race.

Alarmed by the dramatic increase in injuries related to exercise over the past decade, doctors - especially orthopedists - are increasingly voicing their fears that many of the 100 million Americans may be throwing themselves into sports with more zeal than good sense.

Dr. George Sheehan, Cardiologist, confirmed long distance runner, and author of *Running and Living,* states, "If you run, it is not whether you are going to have injuries, it is simply when, and how. You have to be willing to pay the price of blisters, shinsplints, ankle, knee and lower back problems."

Millions of part-time jocks pull muscles, tear cartilages and ligaments, strain tendons, and break their bones each year. Runners lead the pack with not only the highest incidence of injuries but more injuries than are caused by all other recreations combined. This epidemic of strains and sprains is the by-product of the widespread emphasis on aerobic conditioning. This is harmful when it is pursued to the exclusion of other forms of tuning up the rest of the body. A strong cardiovascular system doesn't do much good when the other parts of the body are weak and inflexible.

Today, an estimated 24 million Americans, 90 percent of them women, attend aerobic dance classes convinced that they are perfecting their bodies. But when Peter and Lorna Francis, physical educators at San Diego State University, studied 135 aerobics instructors, they found that 76 percent of the instructors had sustained injuries while teaching their classes. They also found that at least 47 percent of the students get injured. But that percentage may be even higher because often people drop out when they get injured. The type of injuries?

Shin, foot, knee, hip and lower back. Any activity that involves repeated and vigorous pounding of the feet on an unforgiving surface eventually produces some kind of injury. Because of these and other findings, the latest exercise word is low impact aerobics, as opposed to high impact aerobics. If I wait around long enough, our exercise experts will eventually come to the conclusion that rebound exercise (*no impact* aerobics) is "the most efficient, effective form of exercise yet devised by man."

CHAPTER 3

BASIC CONCEPTS OF REBOUND EXERCISE

I want to speak for the Carter family as we look back at the many rich experiences we have had over the last ten years as a direct result of our knowledge of and involvement in rebound exercise. Every day we compare vital information we have learned from the basic concepts of rebound exrcise to outdated information we previously accepted as truths. Even if that was the only benefit we received from rebound exercise, we are truly blessed.

Opposition Necessary to Develop Strength

Ben Yagoda, a frustrated, would-be professional baseball player, if all dreams were allowed to come true, when he was executive editor of *New Jersey Monthly* presented an interesting point of view about jumping in Esquire, November 1981 issue. "Along with running, the jump is probably the athletic activity most elemental to human experience. Consider the expression "jump for joy," or watch a child as he is introduced to a pogo stick or a trampoline, and you'll see what I mean."

But what is jumping? In terms of physics, it is one of the most basic expressions of Newton's law of action and reaction: Pushing down against the ground gives rise to the equal and opposite reaction of being propelled into the air. The power of the jump, according to the science of biomechanics (the science of applying the principles of physics to human movement) is called vertical reaction force (VRF). This is expressed in formula form as $W + ma_y$, where W is the force of gravity on the jumper, m is the body weight (a constant), and a_y is the acceleration.

Important as jumping is to a variety of sports, it is remarkably good exercise in its own right. That's not so surprising when one considers that it may be the purest of athletic endeavors, a simple contest between the jumper and gravity, a willing and constant opponent. This fact was recognized back in 1921 by Dr. Dudley Sargent, who wrote, "I want to share what seems to me the simplest and most effective of all tests of physical ability with the other fools who are looking for one." He then introduced the standing high jump. Apparently this was seen to make sense, for the Sargent Vertical Jump, in which you mark the highest point you can reach and then see how much higher than that you can reach by jumping, is still widely administered in American schools.

Gravity is a Universal Law

Flying across the United States at 37,000 feet, in a very comfortable, climate-controlled, pressurized modern jet plane, I became acutely aware of an interesting fact of my existence. I couldn't see the earth in the darkness of the night, and for the moment, the only thing that existed was the pod in which a few fellow human beings were casually eating, snoozing, reading, and chatting with one another. But our every move was influenced by the same physical force we contend with while we are standing on the earth.

The theory of universal gravitation presented to us by Sir Isaac Newton explains that the same force holding celestial bodies in orbit is also present in the aircraft. That theory states that every element in the universe is subject to the effects of gravity. The moon's gravity pulls on the earth as the earth's pulls on the moon, as evidenced by the moon's influence on the tides as it orbits the earth. Likewise, the liquid in my glass at 37,000 feet pulls as hard on the earth as the earth pulls on the contents of my glass. Now, we live on the earth. Our bodies are primarily affected by the earth's gravitational pull. There are those who believe that a great many people and various species are also influenced by the moon's gravity. Be that as it may, gravity does exist. Newton found that the strength of gravity depends on several things: 1) the amount of matter each body contains; 2) the distance between the bodies. With this information, Newton worked out a formula for the strength of gravity between two bodies:

$$F = \frac{M_1 \times M_2}{R^2}$$

In this equation, if F stands for the force of gravitation. The amount of matter in one body is M_1; amount of matter in the other body is M_2. R is the distance between the bodies.

When distance = 1 $\quad F = \dfrac{M_1 \times M_2}{R^2} = \dfrac{1}{1 \times 1} = 1$

when distance = 2 $\quad F = \dfrac{M_1 \times M_2}{R^2} = \dfrac{1}{2 \times 2} = \dfrac{1}{4}$

when distance = 3 $\quad F = \dfrac{M_1 \times M_2}{R^2} = \dfrac{1}{3 \times 3} = \dfrac{1}{9}$

If the mass of the two bodies remains the same as the

distance doubles, the gravitional pull will be reduced to one-fourth. If the distance between triples, the gravitational pull will be reduced to one-ninth.

On the earth, two other things determine the strength of the gravitational pull: 1) distance from the center of the earth; 2) the spin of the earth. For our purposes, although this difference is measurable, it is not important. Gravity is pulling on all particles of the atmosphere. Therefore, all of us are subjected to the atmospheric pressure. We all live at the bottom of a massive ocean of air that is captured by the gravitational pull of the earth. The weight of the atmosphere is continually fluctuating as a result from air mass motion and changes in the temperature and moisture content of the air.

The device used to measure atmospheric pressure is a barometer, which means, "weight meter." The kind we are most familiar with is a dish filled with mercury into which is inserted a glass tube filled with a vacuum. The weight of the atmosphere presses down on the mercury in the dish and supports a column of mercury inside the tube. At sea level, the pressure of the atmosphere causes the mercury column to rise to almost 30 inches. At five thousand feet above sea level, the atmosphere is only able to support a mercury column about 25 inches high.

Changing altitude, whether in a car or an airplane causes us to swallow several times to allow the pressure to change to the inner ear. But we don't realize that atmospheric pressure dictates the amount of pressure inside our bodies also. It influences every cell throughout the entire body. The pressure inside each cell has to be approximately the same as the pressure on the outside. If too much, the cells will bloat and rupture. If too little, the cells will shrivel. Each cell has the amazing capacity to adjust to the atmospheric pressure we experience on earth. But any time man ventures too far away from the surface of the earth, whether down in the ocean, or to the moon, he must take his environment with him to protect the delicate life of his cells.

Gravity - The Natural Opposition

Therefore, gravity directly influences every cell in the body in two ways: 1) the direct gravitational pull on every individual cell; 2) atmospheric pressure applying pressure from all directions. In fact, Gravity is the most important and constant physical force of our existence. Gravity is one of those laws that were decreed in the Heavens before the foundation of the earth was laid. When we learn to understand and use that law, blessings of health, wisdom and great knowledge are ours for the asking. Now, for all intents and purposes, although gravity is pulling down on everything equally, it has a different effect on living things than on dead, or inanimate objects, like rocks, dirt and fallen leaves. On dead, or non-living things, gravity simply pulls them to their final resting place. But on anything that lives, it provides a force worthy of opposition. You see, the difference between dead things and living things, is that living things have the ability to follow another law just as important and everlasting as gravity. That law? Simply stated: "There must be an opposition in all things to develop strength." Dead things cannot develop strength. Live things can and do. One of the characteristics of all living organisms is their ability to react to changes in their environment. This includes plants, animals, bacteria, human cells, and of course, human beings. But the reason we humans are able to adjust to our environment is because our cells adjust to the environment.

Born into this environment dictated by gravity, we only have two choices: oppose it and become strong; or give up and fold into a compact mass. To surrender to this constant urge, to assume constrictive movements, symbolizes fatigue, withdrawal, defeat and resignation. The catatonic patient who assumes the fetal position is an example of the living refusing to oppose gravity and accepting death.

A newborn baby's first challenge is to lift his head away from the force that is constantly pulling him down.

Gravity, by opposition, becomes the first coach who teaches the baby to crawl, walk, run, jump and play. If not done right, coach Gravity immediately pulls the infant down to try again. This process takes less than a day for a colt, and years for a human baby.

A child starts life with a basic ability to move and a set of distinguishable movement characteristics which are developed during the first three years, specifically with reference to the gravitional forces acting upon the body in relation to the spaces, objects, and surfaces of his environment. Against that constant opposition, the child stands up and becomes an adult.

Man's upright posture governs the way he experiences the world. The vertical and horizontal axes of perceived space are established only with reference to gravity. His visual clues only assist the postural ones. Because the very framework of perceived space is dependent on the need to maintain upright and correct equilibrium against the pull of gravity, the way man sees his world depends on his upright posture. For man to function properly, he must get right with the gravitational pull.

Man's amazing body is designed to achieve equilibrium automatically after the basic procedures are learned. Small sensory hairs in the inner ear are affected by the relationship between gravity and the position and movement of the head. The semi-circular ducts in the inner ear are the sense organs of dynamic equilibrium. They are responsible for initiating body-righting reflexes, making sure that the body is at right angles to the horizontal plane of the earth.

To coordinate body position, there are superficial and deep nerve receptors in the feet and the rest of the body that relay to the control center the relationship of the body to the gravitational force. Impulses from these widely located sensory receptors integrate and converge on a final pathway to bring about effective and coordinated responses of anti-gravity muscles. Strengthening these muscles by proper vigorous exercise enables us to retain or recover normal orientation in space. Equilibrium occurs when we can identify where we are relative to the gravitional pull of the earth.

The expansive, outward movements of a ballet dancer, a gymnast, a trampolinist, or an athlete who seeks to obtain freedom of movement through exercise symbolizes man's aspirations to advance, to rise farther above the earth, to challenge, to live, to achieve, to oppose the downward pull of gravity. When these are achieved, the student has learned his lessons well, all taught by Coach Gravity.

Gravity - The Common Denominator of All Exercise

I am a product of rebound exercise. I started bouncing on a trampoline at fourteen. I won three state championships as an amateur trampolinist. For twelve years, I performed as a professional trampolinist. In 1974 and 1975, my 'Gymnastic Fantastics' professional trampoline team toured the U.S. under the sponsorship of the Marriott Corporation. We criss-crossed the country in our specially equipped motorhome, (shown on the following page) and performed for over half a million people during these two years.

In 1977, I was asked to write an article about the health benefits of jumping on a mini-trampoline-like device. Knowing the health benefits I personally received from trampolining, I accepted the assignment. But I was not willing to write an article without plenty of back-up. The next day, I was in the library checking out books on health, physiology, human anatomy, aerobics and various exercises. Among them were books on trampolining, jogging, jumping rope, and texts on physical education. My concern that day, was locating text books I could quote. I fully expected to find all the information about what happens to the physical body while on the trampoline. After all, hadn't I received this information from my trusted gymnastics instructors? And where had they received their information?

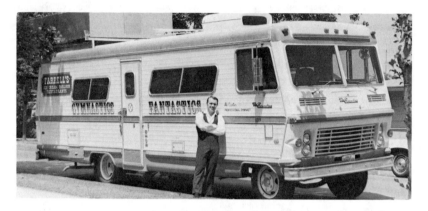

That evening, after the children were in bed, I began to study the stack of books on top of the desk in front of me. Among them was one written by Morehouse, PhD., and Miller M.D., *Physiology of Exercise.* I was immediately impressed with their approach to the subject of exercise and its effect on the health of the human body. On pages 220 and 221, I found activities listed according to the number of calories burned per hour. The list started with sleeping and ended with "horizontal running at 18.9 miles per hour." Imagine my disappointment when I found that trampolining was not among the exercises. Surely, this must be an oversight by the authors. Everyone knows how much energy it takes to bounce on a trampoline. I mean, it is not an unknown. Trampolines have been available to our elementary, junior high, high school, and college students. At one time we had NCAA competition; and even today we have national and world trampoline competition.

I concluded that what I needed in order to write about beneficial bouncing was a physiology with a larger list of exercises. The library had just what I was looking for. I checked out *The International Guide To Fitness And Health*, by Larson and Michelman. Now there's a physiology book! On the front cover it boasted that it was, "from the latest research of the

International Committee on Standardization, which included the fields of medicine, nutrition and physical education . . . the most authoritative techniques for planning a really workable, enjoyable, individual exercise program." Surely this book would have just what I was looking for. I found their activities list beginning on page 50, and it continued for five pages. The exercises were in alphabetical order beginning with archery, and ending with number 133, yard work. It included such activities as "kite flying, putting practice, jai alai, resting, tumbling, and even piloting a plane." But something was missing. Under the T's, I found no mention of trampolining!

Now, I wasn't just disappointed. I was hurt. If I was a baseball player, my sport would be listed. But I'm a trampolinist, and mine wasn't there.

For the next two weeks, I searched *every* library I could find for any physiology books that mentioned trampolining. None. I also pulled out all the books I could find on trampolining written by trampolinists, but to my amazement, even these books made no mention of what actually happens to the body while doing tricks.

In desperation, I finally called the Nissen Corporation in Cedar Rapids, Iowa. Surely they could lead me to the proper resources. After all, according to the *Guinness Book of Records,* it was George Nissen who invented the trampoline in 1936, and it was the Nissen equipment I had been working on for the past twenty years. My call went straight through to the top, and I talked at some length to Bob Bevenour, Executive Vice President. To my dismay, I learned he faced the same problem. He said that he would send me anything that they had in their files, if I would reciprocate by sending any information I found directly to him.

Well, Nissen has been the leader in the trampoline industry for years. If it doesn't have any information of the exercise benefits of trampolining, then I must have been fooling myself all these years. Maybe trampolining was not a better exercise than running. At least it was as good. Discouraged, I decided to write a short page on how running on an "indoor jogger" was a good alternative to outside running. After all, I guess it was rather self-centered of me to imagine that my form of exercise was better than any other.

I was practically sleepless the next week, as I began to return the books to the libraries. Then I began asking myself, "Since trampolining was not included in the lists along with all of the other activities, where would it fit in?"

Rather than returning the last few books, I sat down at a table at the library and began to thumb through the books looking for an answer that didn't seem to be there. I still had an hour before the library closed. I pulled out a piece of paper and began to write down everything all exercises have in common. Halfway through the list, I stopped. I noticed something in common that nobody had even talked about before. I scanned the rest of the exercises. I felt that someone had turned on a light inside my brain.

"That's it!" I exclaimed out loud. I stood up and began to pace around the table, my mind moving a million miles a second trying to recall everything I had read in the last couple of weeks. "It's so simple! Why hasn't anybody thought of it before?"

Please, sir. You are disturbing others." the librarian said approaching me.

"All exercises have one thing in common!" I exclaimed to her. "They are all related to gravity."

"That may be, sir, but we don't exercise in the library. Please be quiet or I'll have to ask you to leave." she said in a not too hushed voice.

"No. Not just related - opposes gravitational pull of the earth. That's it!"

"Sir, are you checking these books in or out?"

"In. No. Out. I have them checked out. I was going to check them in, but now I don't want to. I'll keep them. So I guess neither."

I walked out saying, "The common denominator of all exercises is the opposition to the gravitational pull of the earth!"

In front of the library, I opened the books and went over the exercises one at a time to see if it checked. What about push-ups? Yes, we are pushing away from gravity. Chin-ups? Of course! And Sit-ups? Gravity is pulling on our torso as we pull away from the floor. Leg-lifts? We are opposing gravity with the other ends of our bodies. What about weight lifting? Sure. the word, "weight" by definition is "mass times gravity."

Even the aerobic exercises fit into the category. To walk, you first move your center of gravity in the direction you wish to go until you start falling that direction. Then you take a series of steps to keep from falling. Jogging and running are accomplished by allowing gravity to pull down on the upper body longer before taking steps to recover. Walking, jogging, and running are simply a state of continuous falling almost, but not quite catching your balance until you decide to stop.

Dancing is falling in various directions while overcompensating at various steps to change direction and control the rhythm of the fall.

Even swimming is directly influenced by the gravitational pull of the earth. Although the body appears to be defying the law of gravity by floating, keep in mind that floating is not an exercise. Swimming is. It is the downward pull of gravity on the molecules of the water which make water dense enough to establish resistance to the muscles of the swimmer.

Every exercise listed was functional as an exercise because of its demand of energy in opposing gravity - even trampolining - and it wasn't listed among the exercises.

Albert Einstein's Contribution to the Ideal Exercise

During the next few weeks, my patient wife, Bonnie, and I spent every spare moment, and even some we couldn't spare, writing and rewriting the manuscript of *Rebound to Better*

Health. The book began to take shape; arguments were labored, but, we felt, convincing. However, there was still something missing. We knew there had to be something more than just opposing gravity, but we couldn't quite put our fingers on it. Finally, after several nights of writing and rewriting, we came to a fatigued and dismal halt.

One night, after midnight, I was alone at my desk. I felt trapped by my commitment and not able to do anything about it. "Oh God, what are we not seeing?" I prayed. I went to a set of encyclopedias, the *New Book of Knowledge,* and looked up "gravity" on page 320 in volume 7. Gloom descended as I read:

"For 300 years scientists have studied gravitation. They can measure its strength and tell other things about it, but the question, 'What is gravitation?' is still a mystery."

I continued to read:

"In 1911, the famous scientist, Albert Einstein, developed a new idea of gravitation. He showed that gravitation, acceleration, and deceleration produced the same effects. There is no way to tell gravitation from acceleration or deceleration."

I looked up from the book in a half-daze. "That's it!" I said aloud. "That's what's missing! Bonnie. Bonnie, we've found it!"

I leaped from my chair, grabbed the book and tripped up the stairs to our bedroom where Bonnie lay sleeping.

"I found the key! I found what we've been looking for, and it's been in our basement all the time!"

"You found what?" she asked, trying to come awake.

"The key." I exclaimed, out of breath.

"I didn't know we had lost one."

"Listen, there is more than one force we are working with!"

"Let's talk about it in the morning," she said, rolling over and pulling the covers over head.

"How can you sleep when I'm so excited?"

"I can't. So I'll listen," she said, sitting up. "Now, what did you find in our basement?"

"The answer explaining why rebounding is so much better than all other exercises!

"We've been talking about opposing gravity. All exercises do that, but acceleration and deceleration are two completely different forces. Although they're different, the human body can't tell the difference. Therefore, if you accelerate vertically like in a rocketship or on a trampoline, you develop a greater G force."

"Oh, I get it." she brightened, "If you come down and stop, you decelerate and for just a moment the body feels the combined effects of deceleration and gravity, and responds like somebody had suddenly turned up the earth's gravitational pull."

"Right. And where do all three of these forces come together for just a moment?"

"At the bottom of the bounce?" she asked, timidly.

"Exactly. That is why I can still do over one hundred one-arm push-ups although I have never lifted weights. My entire body has adjusted to a greater G force environment than the normal G force everyone else experiences here on the earth."

"If that's the case, all trampolinists have extra unexplained strengths."

"Right. Who do we know who are trampolinists?"

"Our children. Both Darren and Wendie have been on the trampoline since before they could walk."

"That explains why Darren was able to do 429 sit-ups the first time he was challenged, even though he's only in the first grade."

"And why Wendie was able to beat him at 476 sit-ups without stopping. And why she was able to beat all of the sixth grade boys in arm wrestling even though she had never arm wrestled in her life."

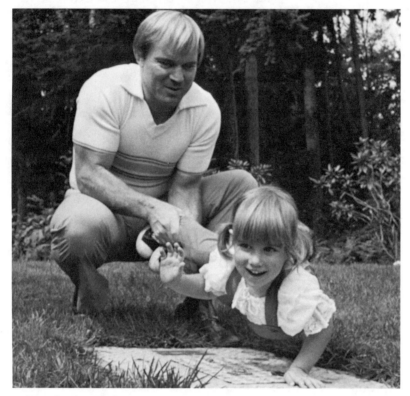

"And why Melynda can do 'one-arm pushups' at age 3½."

For the next two hours, we brainstormed, and things began to fall into place.

The next day, I researched *Medical Physiology* by Arthur C. Guyton. The chapter entitled "Space Physiology" verified what we had discovered. It pointed out that the federal government had already spent millions investigating the effects of acceleration and deceleration on our astronauts both horizontally and vertically. However, those studies were designed to see how much G force the body could stand without physical damage or blacking out, not how much was needed to enhance health.

One thing is sure. The forces of acceleration and deceleration do exist. We don't have to pay for them. They are ours. Free. so let's look at them.

Acceleration Another Force

When we want to go someplace, we get in our automobile and step on the accelerator. The increasing speed of the forward motion of the automobile pushes us back into the seat. A gun kicks because of the reaction of the acceleration of the bullet. Test pilots were strapped into jet sleds that ran across the desert on rails. The sleds were allowed to accelerate so fast that the men experienced a G force nine or ten times that of gravity. This was necessary to find out if the astronauts would be able to withstand the seven G force during lift-off at Cape Kennedy. That G force meant that a 175 pound astronaut would weigh 1225 pounds immediately after blast off.

Deceleration - Yet Another Force

In a moving automobile, if we want to slow down or stop, we apply the brake, or the decelerator. We experience the force of deceleration. A carpenter drives a nail when the force of deceleration of the head of the hammer is expended against the head of the nail. When the astronauts returned to earth, they experienced another increase in their body weight during the deceleration part of their re-entry flight. Huge drag-parachutes opened to slow their landing module during re-entry into the earth's atmosphere, and their bodies increased in weight by at least 4½ G's. One of the G forces was gravity, but the other 3½ Gs were deceleration. However, their bodies accepted this change the same as an increase in gravity.

I felt the force of acceleration when my Boeing jet began to increase to flight speed as it rolled down the runway for take off. Although I was trying to lean forward to look out the window, the acceleration force pushed me back into my seat.

When the plane touched down, my body strained against the seat belt until we had slowed sufficiently to turn and taxi to our gate.

It is really strange to me that although our space scientists have studied the effects of these forces on our bodies, they haven't used this information to develop a space-age exercise. Sometimes the simplicity of an idea completely mystifies our scientists, but is easily understood by the common man.

I was explaining the rebound concept to an audience in Pennsylvania when an Amish gentleman stood up and said, "Mr. Carter, what you are trying to tell us is that we have three natural forces available to us at no cost that we should use to exercise effectively, but we haven't been harnessing them up right."

"What do you mean?" I asked.

"Well, it is as if I had three powerful horses hooked up to one plow with one pulling to the right, one pulling to the left, and one pulling straight ahead. I would have a hard time plowing my field, wouldn't I?"

"You have the idea exactly," I said. We have accepted the forces of acceleration and deceleration as parts of our environment because they exist, but we haven't considered even for a moment the combined therapeutic impact of these forces on the human body. We know they exist. We know that everybody has to cope with them. But what's the most efficient way to use them? Obviously, our Amish farmer will get more plowing done by making sure all three horses pull in the same direction. So, by lining up acceleration and deceleration with gravity in the same direction, it stands to reason that these forces have a greater impact on the body.

The Vertical Stacking of Natural Forces

The gravitational force pulling on everything on this earth is vertical. We cannot change that. As long as we live here on Mother Earth, we are subject to gravity and we cannot control it. However, we can control the direction and intensity of the forces of velocity, acceleration and deceleration. A baseball pitcher depends upon his ability to accelerate the pitched baseball to between seventy and a hundred miles an hour in a horizontal direction towards the home plate. The batter's objective is to accelerate the bat in the opposite direction sufficient to cause the ball to, first, decelerate to a complete stop for a split second, then to accelerate in the approximate direction to a velocity capable of carrying it out of the ball park before gravity captures it. A catcher uses his mitt to decelerate the ball when the batter misses it. Although these forces have been in existence ever since mass was acted upon by force, we have never considered them as viable tools when it comes to exercising the body. For example. Have you ever heard a physical education instructor yell, "Come on you guys, accelerate ten more times!" or, "Let's get out there and decelerate twenty times."

The most efficient and effective way to harness these untrapped forces is to line them up with gravity. That's the purpose of the rebounder. As you stand still on the rebounder, every cell in your body is subject to the force of gravity. This can be measured with a "G" meter. Are you familiar with a "G" meter? You probably have a "G" meter in your own home. You call it a bathroom scale. If you were to put a bathroom scale on top of a rebounder and stand on it, it would register the amount of G force the earth was pulling down on your entire body. One G force would be your total weight. However, something fascinating happens when you start moving up and down. You begin to subject your entire body to the forces of acceleration and deceleration, plus gravity. At the bottom of the bounce, your whole body stops. That's deceleration. Then, it increases in speed upward. That's acceleration. The combination of vertical deceleration followed instantly by vertical acceleration of your entire body combining with the constant gravity creates an increased G force which is felt by every cell in your body. You no longer weigh 1 G, you weigh more! The cells react to this environmental stimulation the same way they react to any other environmental change. They adjust by becoming individually stronger. When your feet leave the mat, your body begins to slow down. Deceleration again. When you start down, you accelerate until your feet sink into the mat enough to cause the springs to slow you down. Your whole body feels the effect of acceleration and deceleration an average of two hundred times a minute! What effects does this exert on your body? Let me explain at least three.

At the bottom of the bounce, every cell in your body identifies the combination of the three forces simply as an increase in the gravitational pull of the earth, much the same way they would react if they experienced your living on a larger planet than the earth with a greater G force. This happens a hundred times a minute!

At the top of the bounce, as gravity counteracts the combined forces of the change in velocity, you become weightless for a fraction of a second a hundred times a minute. All cells of your body immediately become weightless. Virtually all immediate structural stresses and pressure are eliminated from all of your cells all at once.

Your cells depend upon the diffusion of water through their semi-permeable cell membranes (the outside surface of the cell) to carry oxygen, nutrients, hormones, enzymes into the cell, and to flush out metabolic trash. The rate of diffusion of water into and out of the cells under normal conditions is 100 times the volume of fluid inside each cell each second. The oscillation of the cells of your body between an increase in G force and a no G force 200 times a minute increases the diffusion of water into each cell at least three fold! Nothing beats that kind of cellular cleansing.

CHAPTER 4

REBOUNDING:
THE WHOLE-BODY EXERCISE

Suddenly we have been catapulted from the old-fashioned inefficient methods of exercising we have all been taught for the last fifty years. Calisthenics, weight lifting and jogging, exercise only part of the body at a time by isolating muscle groups and providing an exercise designed for that particular group. We have come face-to-face with a whole-body exercise. To be more precise, rebounding is a cellular exercise because it causes all of the cells of the body to physically adjust to what is perceived by them as a more demanding internal environment. We didn't ask their permission. We just did it. They have to adjust.

NASA Studies Rebounding

It's crazy, but it works," said C. E. (Pat) Mueller, director of recreational sports at the University of Minnesota for thirty years. "I've seen a lot of sports fads come and go," said Mueller, an associate professor with a master's degree in physical education. "But this thing is so phenomenal — It's the exercise

37

of the future.

Rebounding has been around for over fifty years. What's new is our understanding of rebound exercise as a process of gravitational force overloading."

Professor Pat Mueller is the one who brought my attention to the NASA Report published in the *Journal of Applied Physiology* 49(5): 881-887, 1980, which confirms many of the statements previously made in the first printing of *"The Miracles of Rebound Exercise".* The research was performed by the Biomechanical Research Division, NASA-Ames Research Center, Moffett Field, California, in cooperation with the Wenner-Gren Research Laboratory, University of Kentucky, Lexington.

The four scientists, A. Bhattacherya, E. P. McCutcheon, E. Shavartz, and J. E. Greenleaf, secured the assistance of eight young men between the ages of 19 and 26, requiring each to walk, jog and run on a treadmill operated at four different speeds, and then jump on a standard-sized trampoline at four different heights in order to compare the difference between the two modes of exercise. Although treadmill running had been studied many times before, the scientists found that ". . . measurements of the necessary variables have not been reported previously for trampoline exercise." A Summary of that study is found in the back of this book, but there are a few quotes that seem to fit here.

". . . for similar levels of heart rate and oxygen consumption, the magnitude of the biomechanical stimuli is greater with jumping on a trampoline than with running, a finding that might help identify acceleration parameters needed for the design of remedial procedures to avert deconditioning in persons exposed to weightlessness."

"The external work output at equivalent levels of oxygen uptake were significantly greater while trampolining than running. The greatest difference was about 68%. Now, if you had access to a gasoline that was 68% more efficient than the gasoline you are using in your automobile right now at the same price, wouldn't you take advantage of it? Well, we don't have the gasoline, but it does appear that we do have the exercise.

It is fitting that NASA should explore trampolining, or, as we know it now, rebound exercise, because they had a real need for an exercise breakthrough. They found that when the astronauts were sent into space, in as little as fourteen days they lost as much as 15% of their bone and muscle mass. The space rats didn't do as well. In seven days, their loss was as much as 40%.

It appears that the cells of the body have a greater ability to adjust to their environment than we give them credit for. Without gravity, the cells of the bones and muscles took it upon themselves to adjust. Strong bones are not necessary in a zero gravity environment, so the osteocytes (bone cells) become osteoclasts and began to dissolve bone mineral from the bones. (Medical doctors know that when bones are stressed, the bone cells perform osteoblastic activity by absorbing bone mineral and depositing it in the bones where they are being stressed.)

Did NASA find their space age exercise? It appears so. Rebounding appears to be a way of "...averting the deconditioning that occurs during the immobilization of bed rest of space flight, due to a lack of gravireceptor stimulation (in addition to other factors)." [Recovering from space flight] "...requires an acceleration profile that can be delivered at a relatively low metabolic cost." Their studies pointed out that "While trampolining, as long as the G-force remained below 4-G's, the ratio of oxygen consumption compared to biomechanical conditioning was sometimes more than twice as efficient as treadmill running."

It is important to note that although this experiment was performed on a trampoline where the participants were able to develop a G-force as high as 8-G's, the efficient use of energy was below 4-G's.

That brings up two immediate questions. 1) What is the maximum G-force that can be developed on a rebounder? and 2) How much G-force can an average person handle? In other words, is rebounding really safe for the normal person? We need to call in the United States Air Force to answer that question. USAF pilots have been pulling multi-G's ever since it's existence.

The Air Force Studies Rebounding

I first met Maj. Ward Dean, M.D., United States Air Force, over the telephone. He had just read *The Miracles of Rebound Exercise,* and decided that he didn't like some of the things I had said. His major complaint was that I was making statements that were not supported by scientific studies and documentation. "Sure, I can handle criticism," I remember saying. He then spent the next ninety minutes telling me what was wrong with my book. Personally, I was devastated. That telephone conversation left me weak. To make things worse, I received a letter a week later enumerating the many fallacies of my work. I did study his suggestions and corrected the mistakes of the book during subsequent printings.

I was surprised one day when Dr. Dean called me and asked me what he could test in his laboratory in Korea. I suggested that he establish how many G's a person could develop on a rebounder. "Okay." He said, "It's as good as done."

Near the end of January, 1983, I received a copy of his Master's Thesis for his Master's Degree in Physiology from Kyungbook University, College of Medicine in Taegu, Korea. The subject? How much G force can be developed by an athlete in good physical condition bouncing on a quality rebounder at maximum attainable altitude. His scientific conclusions are 3.24 G's.

In a chapter of *Medical Physiology*, entitled, Space Physiology, Guyton points out that the normal human can handle as much as 8 Gs momentarily, and 20 Gs in a sitting position before vertebral fracture occurs. If the transverse acceleration forces are applied uniformly over large areas of the body, as much as 15 to 25 Gs can be withstood. The point being, that if the best athletes can develop only 3.24 Gs, rebounding is a safe whole body-exercise for virtually every body.

The University of Utah Studies Rebounding

I guess the question of safety has to be an important one, especially since every book on exercise has one or two chapters on injury, everything from dog bites to shin splints. This is probably what prompted Craig McQueen, M.D., to ask A. W. Daniels, Ph.D., Adjunct Professor, Material Science and Engineering and Orthopedic Surgery of the University of Utah to analyze the comparison of the impact loads transmitted by rebounding and more conventional exercise surfaces.

In this report, they compared rebounding to jogging. Briefly, they accomplished the following:

Determined the approximate spring constant of the rebounder by measuring the deflection of the surface when various persons of known weight stood on it. It was found that the constant was 770 lb/ft.

Calculated the length of time of impulse load contact for a "typical" 165 lb. person running on a rebounder, and on a wooden board track where the constant was 33,000 lb/ft. The time of contact is inversely proportional to the impact force. The calculated times of contact were .13 seconds for the rebounder and .02 seconds on the wooden board track.

Since .02 is only about 15% of the .13, the maximum impact force on the rebounder would be only 1/6th that of the wooden board track.

One of the major problems runners have is structural damage caused by the constant pounding of the skeleton against unforgiving surfaces.

Peter Daetwiler of Hong Kong, an executive of a hotel chain, was a runner who needed weekly cortisone shots in his knee to combat the pain and swelling before he was turned on to rebound exercise. He was then able to maintain his level of cardiovascular endurance in the safety and convenience of his home in less time, and without the expensive and painful medication.

Dr. Harry Sneider Studies Rebounding

"I know how to make rebound exercise even better," I heard one day when I was at the National Health Federation Convention, in Anaheim, California. The voice belonged to Harry Sneider, fitness coach of Ambassador College, in Pasadena, California.

"If you can improve on rebound exercise, you have my

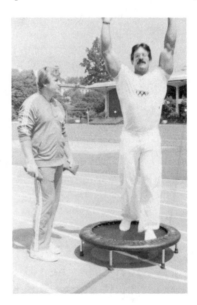

Dr. Harry Sneider introduces Mr. Universe, 1979, Mike Kentzer to Aerobic Resistive Rebounding.

undivided attention," I remember saying. That was the beginning of Aerobic Resistive Rebounding, a simple concept of putting light weights in the hands and running, jumping or bouncing on a rebounder while moving the weights in organized motions. Since Harry Sneider's background was that of training body builders and training athletes for Olympic competition, he felt rebounding would fit in his system of honing and fine-tuning his athletes. The cellular, or whole-body exercise concept was appealing to him, but he wasn't going to turn his back on resistance training. It took a little ingenuity and 1, 2, and 3 pound sand bags to combine the two exercise methods. This is one case where the sum of the two parts is greater than the parts.

Resistive, on isotonic exercise, involves muscle contraction under opposition with movement. Weight lifting is a good

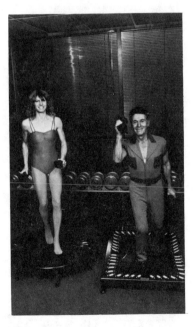

Sarah Sneider joins Jack LaLane in an Aerobic Resistive Rebounding Exercise workout.

example of organized resistive exercise. Who can argue with success? I am not about to argue with Mr. Universe or Jack Lalanne, but when Dr. Sneider began to introduce rebound exercise to them, they too caught on to the fun and easy benefits.

Engineers Study Rebound Exercise

One way exercise is measured is by the amount of work performed, or accomplished. So I turned the problem over to an engineer friend of mine. I introduced him to *Harry and Sarah Sneider's Olympic Trainer,* an exercise package consisting of three sets of hand-held weights, 1, 2, and 3 pound sandbags to be used in conjunction with rebounding. The participant goes through an organized series of upper body movements while walking, jumping or running on a rebounder. His conclusions are simple but revealing. He has been kind enough to take us through easy-to-understand logical steps to an amazing conclusion. You'll enjoy the step by step logic.

Step 1. If one stands still on the rebounder and holds a one pound weight in each hand, it will exert one pound pressure on each arm, a total of two pounds on the trunk and legs.

See? that's easy to understand. If you stand on a bathroom scales and somebody hands you two pounds of butter, the scales will add two pounds to your weight.

Step 2. If one jumps on a rebounder creating a 2 G force, the weight will create 2 pounds of force at the bottom of the bounce on each arm; a total of 4 pounds on the trunk and legs.

Your weight is doubled when you bounce high enough to create 2 Gs. Even your clothes weigh twice as much. Even the weights in your hands weigh twice as much.

Step 3. If one creates the bounce by rhythmically moving the weights in the hands forcefully up and down, the G force is at least doubled again at the

bottom of the bounce and 1 G of deceleration at the top of the bounce. This subjects each arm to an additional five pounds of resistance, or a total of 10 pounds.

If you are analyzing this as we go, you are beginning to see the synergistic effects of two forms of exercise being combined into one.

Step 4. If one moves the weights from the shoulders to the waist while sinking into the mat six inches and bouncing off the mat six inches, the weights in the hands move upward a total of approximately 2 feet each bounce.

Remember, the formula for work-produced is weight-times-distance.

Step 5. Assume one bounces six inches off the mat 100 times in a minute, moving the weights 1 foot in a curl exercise. That would be moving 10 pounds x 2 feet x 100 times, or 2000 foot/pounds of work in one minute. . . . or, if you used 2 pound weights with the same exercise, it would be 4000 foot/pounds of work. . . . or, if you used the three pound weights, 6000 foot/pounds.

That's three tons of work! The skeptic will say, "That's impossible," then go out and lift one-forth of his automobile with a small jack in order to fix a flat.

Step 6. For the purpose of illustration, let's assume that you use the two pound weights moving them an average of one foot while sinking six inches into the mat and bouncing six inches off the mat. You complete the Daily Dozen (a series of exercises shown in "Harry and Sarah Sneider's Olympic Trainer"), 25 repetitions, 3 sets. It takes you 20 minutes. This would be the equivalent of moving a 40 ton freight car 1 foot in 20 minutes, or a Volkswagen up 40 steps in 20

**minutes, or curling a 100 pound barbell 200 times
in 20 minutes!**

That's just calculating the movement of the weights in your
hands, what about your body?

**Step 7. Assume you weigh 150 pounds and are
bouncing high enough to create 2 Gs. At the
bottom of the bounce you weigh 300 pounds. Your
entire weight is moved upward 1 foot 100 times
a minute x 20 minutes, or 600,000 foot/pounds!**

That's the equivalent of moving a 300 ton freight train engine
1 foot in 20 minutes! Add that to the 40 ton freight car and
you will begin to understand why resistive rebounding is
destined to revolutionize our concept of weight training.
Granted, the springs in the rebounder do some of the work,
but that's the beauty of it. Your cells can't tell the difference!

Dr. Kenneth Cooper's Institute of Aerobics Research Studies Rebounding

Anything as amazing as the reported results of rebound
exercise doesn't stay hidden forever. Those who begin to enjoy
the benefits become disciples. They extol the virtues of
rebounding, and soon even the most skeptical come around.
Scientists are skeptics by profession. Somebody sent copies
of my *"Miracles"* and *"Sneider's Olympic Trainer"* to Dr.
Kenneth Cooper's Institute of Aerobics Research in Dallas,
Texas. Near the end of 1981, I received a telephone call from
R. Donald Hagan, Ph.D, Director of Exercise Physiology, telling
me that some of the stories in the *"Miracles"* were simply too
hard to believe. When I told him that they were all true, he
asked me, "Are they backed by scientific studies?"

"No." I said. "I'm not a scientist. I'm merely reporting what
I'm learning."

"Well, we need scientific evidence before we can accept
rebound exercise as a viable form of exercise."

"You're a scientist aren't you?" I countered. "Why don't you study rebound exercise and report back to me? Besides, it will be more credible if you perform the study rather than us." I received a letter dated December 10, 1981, confirming our conversation, which began, "It has been a pleasure talking to you about rebound exercise. We are preparing a research proposal to study rebound exercise... We would be most interested in evaluating the 'daily dozen charts' outlined in Dr. Sneider's book on rebounding, and any other exercise program that you believe people would be interested in knowing about."

The report of the completed study came across my desk six months later. They must have been impressed because this is the way it started out:

The Institute of Aerobics Research Study
NEW SUPER CIRCUIT PROGRAM
conditions the whole body for
endurance, strength and flexibility

"These findings will have significant impact at every level of physical conditioning, whether in high school, college, professional team sports medicine, or fitness programs.

Super Circuit will help move participants through their conditioning program faster, with greater overall conditioning effectiveness. And, it will provide much of the needed aerobic conditioning for their particular sports without subjecting their bodies to lifting very heavy weights or jogging great distances in a running program.

This was the fifth study Dr. Larry Gettman, Ph.D, Paul Ward, Ph.D, and R.D. Hagan Ph.D, had undertaken to examine the cardiorespiratory aspects of isokinetic and isotonic weight training. It lasted twelve weeks and consisted of 36 females

and 41 males reflecting the average condition of normally active people. The difference between the Super Circuit group and the control group was that those who participated in the Super Circuit rebounded for 30 seconds in between each of the circuit weight training stations.

These Super Circuit aerobic results are the highest ever reported in circuit weight training scientific literature...But the Super Circuit has other advantages, too. There is less skeletal shock and joint stress..., plus, strength gains showed a 25% improvement over the standard circuit weight training!"

Strength gains are important, especially for those who are looking for strength, but the most important aspect was the lack of skeletal shock as pointed out earlier by the study at the University of Utah. So, who needs this information?

The Need for Rebound Aerobics in Professional Exercise Facilities

"Thousands of Bouncing, Bopping Aerobic Enthusiasts May Be Doing Themselves Grave Bodily Harm."

So began an article in *People Magazine,* June 2, 1986. They quoted Jane Fonda in her 1981 Workout Book, "You must work hard, sweat hard, and get sore." Millions followed her advice and now, according to the latest studies, they may be badly harming themselves.

Today, an estimated 24 million Americans, 90% of them women, jump through steps and stretches on hard floors doing what is known as Aerobic Dance. Peter and Lorna Francis, physical educators at San Diego State University, studied 135 aerobic instructors and found that 75% of them had sustained injuries. The injuries were shin, foot, knee, hip and lower back. "Any activity that involves repeated and vigorous pounding of the feet on the unforgiving ground produces some kind of injury. . ."

It is estimated that 43% of the students are injured, but this percentage may be higher because often people drop out when they get hurt. However, the blame is not totally that of the instructor, because most instructors are self taught. At health clubs, they work at a very high intensity. Many between the ages of 21 and 25 feel that abuse is good for them. Often the students demand a hard, driving session, and the instructors are afraid they will lose their clientele or their job if they conduct a more moderate exercise. The instructor has the responsibility of a fitness coach without the experience, and the students suffer. Very few will argue that Jane Fonda is not an attractive lady, but she's not an exercise expert. As a result, we have the blind leading the blind leading the blind. It has only been in the last few years that aerobics dance instructors are able to have training or be licensed. Where do we go from here? We have a solution.

Aerobics Club Bounces Into Fitness and Profits

An Olympia, Washington fitness center found it literally bounced back from a slump in student interest caused by the bad press on high impact aerobics.

The student's acceptance of aerobic routines on rebounders was enthusiastic. The floor space limited the classes to 30 students, and the demand required them to reserve their units in advance.

"Rebounding is perfect for a 40-minute class. After a few weeks, the members start to see major improvements in their bodies," Ms. Martin said. "There haven't been any injuries, and those people who start with the classes stay with them."

She explained that the students are able to work through and rehabilitate old injuries and back problems caused by previous aerobic routines. With the use of the rebounders, they were able to strengthen and tone their bodies while reducing the impact by approximately 87%.

"The entire industry is changing to focus on less injury. We find there's a big interest in low impact aerobics. Rebounding is a specialty we can offer, and some people come here because of it," the studio owner said.

From the student's standpoint, rebounding is the answer to the problem of previous injuries or daily pressures.

"There is high-impact, low-impact and rebounding, which is virtually no-impact aerobics," describes Lucinda Baker. A rebound enthusiast for more than a year, she found the exercise easy on her body, especially after recently having a child.

"It's perfect for controlling the stomach, particularly when I don't have time to do weight training," she said. She first noticed the lost inches on her stomach and hips, but found other areas also benefit.

"I had many injuries from running marathons," explained John Phillips, who said that his exercise had been limited to weight training. "Before rebounding I just couldn't do any type of movement exercise. Now those foot problems I had for several years are a thing of the past."

For more information on the ProBounder 2000 Contact:
NEW DIMENSIONS DISTRIBUTORS
16548 E. Laser Drive
Fountain Hills, Arizona 85268
Call 1-800-624-7114 Toll-Free Nationwide
In Arizona (602) Call: 1-837-8322

CHAPTER 5

REBOUNDING: FAD? FANTASY? FICTION? OR, INDUSTRY?

What's in a name? Parents, please pay particular attention to the name you select for your children. A handle is vitally important to any person, place, or thing. I have a confession to make. When I went to Snohomish (pronounced, snow-ho-mish) Publishing Company in 1978, to talk to them about printing the first 10,000 *Miracles,* I had written an introduction describing myself on the inside front cover. It said: "Washington State's foremost authority on rebound exercise." "Now, I thought that was pretty bold, but since I was writing my own book, somebody had to say something good about the author if we were going to sell any copies at all.

Bill Bates, the co-owner of Snohomish Publishing, and my editor, asked me why I made such a claim.

"Because I don't know of anybody in the state of Washington that knows any more about Rebound Exercise, " I said in defense.

"Do you know of anybody in the United States who has such a grasp on rebounding?" he asked.

51

"No. Because I am the only trampolinist who has both experienced rebounding and then studied it enough to write a book on the subject."

"Do you know anyone in the whole world who understands rebounding as you do?"

"No."

"Then why stop at the State of Washington?"

Thus, I carry the distinction of being the World's foremost authority on "the most efficient, effective form of exercise yet devised by man" - rebound exercise.

I walked away from Snohomish Publishing with a new handle - a heavy handle. In that instant my life changed, never to be the same again. To me, to be world's foremost authority on anything was quite an accomplishment. To be honest, I felt a little guilty because I hadn't really worked that hard for such a title. It reminded me of when, in my freshman year in high school, I placed third in the Montana State Wrestling Championships - quite an accomplishment, right? Today, it would be, but that year there were only three wrestlers in my weight class who went to the state meet! I didn't tell anyone how stiff my competition was, but being second runner up made me work much harder the next year. I took the Montana State Wrestling Championship in my sophomore year - and I earned it!

As I left Snohomish that day, I realized it might be but for a fleeting moment in the history of mankind that I was truly the world's foremost authority until I was challenged by someone who possessed greater knowledge about rebound exercise. But I had already made up my mind that I was going to be ready for that challenge when it did come. Because I had no way of knowing who else was studying rebound exercise, what their background was, or how much time they were able to spend on the subject each day, I became a fanatic. Every waking moment was spent on searching for more ways rebounding could enhance the health of the human body.

However, a curious thing happened. Those who read the book just seemed to accept my precarious position without question. Or at least, nobody wanted it for himself enough to attempt to lay claim on my title. Rather than challenge me, they seemed quite content to refer to me as the authority. That way, they didn't have to bear the burden of making bold statements that couldn't be backed up by some other authority.

In the latter part of 1979, we incorporated *The National Institute of Reboundology and Health, Inc.* Our initial intent was to have the Institute publish my books. But in less than six months, it had grown beyond our wildest expectations. There was such a need for information about rebound exercise that people from all over the world began to ask us major health and fitness questions simply because there was nowhere else to turn.

Certified Reboundologists - The Professional Bouncer

One day, my wife and I were in downtown Seattle driving by the Seattle Center, the site of the '64 World's Fair, when we noticed a blinking neon sign informing the world of the science of *"Mixology"* the study of mixing drinks - a bartending school. I remarked to Bonnie, "Since I have been studying a new form of exercise, it could be called *"Reboundology."* We both laughed at the funny sounding word.

"That's terrible," exclaimed Bonnie, "Because you would be called a *"Reboundologist."* Again we broke out in laughter.

"And when we teach rebound exercise to professionals, they would be *"Certified Reboundologists"!* Again we laughed, but this time the laughter died away into serious thought. Before the next exit on the freeway, we both came to the same conclusion. We took that exit and went back to talk to our attorney.

"Sure, you can protect the terms *Reboundology* and *Reboundologist*. And while you're at it, you might as well protect *Certified Reboundologist,"* he advised.

"Great!" We said in unison. "What do we have to do to protect the terms?"

"Simple. Produce one."

"Pardon?"

"To protect a new term, you need to define it by production. You need to develop a Certified Reboundologist, other than yourself, by writing a study manual and developing a training seminar whereby those who desire can become Certified by the National Institute of Reboundology and Health, Inc., as a Professional Reboundologist. Then, all you have to do is sell the seminar and provide the certification after they have met the requirements set forth by the Institute."

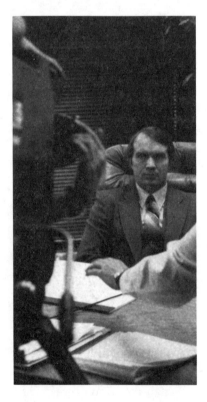 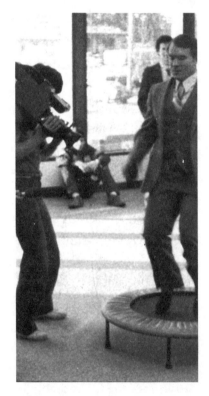

A TV shoot at the Institute

We began immediately to write, plan and develop a course whereby people could be certified. Our first three-day Reboundology Seminar was held early in 1981 at the Sheraton Plaza, in Los Angeles, followed immediately by another one in Amarillo, Texas.

Successful? Judge for yourself. Following are statements of people who became Certified Reboundologists in those two seminars.

"I feel that the time and effort I spent here was well spent. It opened up a whole new way of thinking for me. . ." *LeGrande Rane,* San Diego, CA.

"Fantastic! Fantastic! Fantastic! Everyone should attend, if only for their own information!" - *Irvin Widmer,* McBride, B.C. Canada

"I would recommend this course to anyone who desires to put the puzzle of body, mind, and spirit completely together with the catalyst, cellular exercise." - *Liz Rothwell,* Rancho Cordova, CA.

"After six years of 'rebounding', this course helped make logical and physiological clarity of what I thought was happening. An excellent, non-traditional compendium of information concerning this remarkable form of exercise and education. I found it most worthwhile." - *J. Patrick Netter,* Los Angeles.

"The Reboundology Seminar has been more informative than any other exercise class I have participated in. Most of my friends would be interested in rebounding because the concept teaches why it makes you feel better." - *Sandi Bannister,* Amarillo, TX.

I could go on and on, because there are now approximately one thousand Certified Reboundologists in the World!

NIRH - The Rebound Information Magnet

One of the benefits I didn't first consider is the preponderance of information Reboundologists would send into the Institute.

With hundreds of enthused people aware of cellular exercise, every time something was published in any newspaper or magazine, either to support our position or refute it, I received half a dozen copies across my desk. The Institute became a magnet for any information about rebound exercise. It isn't hard to maintain my position as the "World's Foremost Authority of Rebound Exercise" when I'm constantly receiving the latest information on my chosen subject.

So, what did we talk about in the Reboundology Seminars? I was told by a marketing and advertising agency that the rebound industry was like a diamond in the rough. Everytime we polished a facet, we found another one next to it just as bright. Each one of the following subjects is being expanded to another book, so they will be treated only in summary here.

Rebounding - A Cellular Exercise

This claim is fantastic when you really think about it. But is it really true? It became necessary for me to become intimately familiar with the cells of the body. Although the human body is made up of seventy-five trillion cells, each requiring approximately the same environment and same nutrients, there are about two-hundred different types of cells.

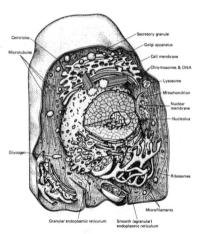

All cells have a cell membrane, the outer surface; cytoplasm, the inside; and a nucleus, the management part of the cell. Now, we all know that, or we should, because this is what we learned in school. We also learned that a cell is like a busy city. In fact, as one doctor explained to me at five-thousand feet over

Chicago, "Look as far as you can see in all directions. Imagine you are aware of every type of movement in the city regardless of where it is. As soon as you can comprehend all that activity, you will have an idea of the amount of activity going on inside each cell of your body."

The cell membrane of each cell has to be strong enough to keep from rupturing under normal environmental conditions, but flexible enough to allow movement. Therefore, all cells have a rupture threshold which is controlled internally by enzymes (minute molecular factory workers) which have the responsibility of monitoring the strength of the cell membrane. When the membrane is challenged in any way, the enzyme sends a message to the DNA, which sends a message to the ribosomes, the molecular factories responsible for making structural proteins. Enzymes then transport the proteins to the cell membrane and install them, making the membrane stronger. The structural strength of the cell membrane is directly related to the environmental stresses placed upon the cells. At low Gs, the membrane becomes weak. At high Gs, the cells become stronger.

The Mitrochondria - The Energy to Burn

A part of the cell we usually don't hear about is the powerhouse, or mitrochondria. Without them, the cells would

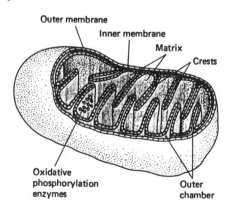

not be able to function because they are the source of all the energy the cells need to import nutrients, export waste products, and manu- facture hormones, carry on other cellular activities, and contract. This high energy substance is called *adenosine triphosphate*

(ATP). ATP is transported out of the mitochondria and diffused throughout the cell to release its energy wherever it is needed for performing cellular functions.

Besides being the energy source for lighting us up, another important factor is that the mitochondria have the ability to replicate themselves whenever their energy is used up. This means that one can form two, then three whenever there is a need for increased amounts of energy. Why is this so important? Simply because with a cellular exercise, like rebounding, all of the cells begin using energy, more powerhouses are produced and the entire body has more energy to burn. This is why a person who starts rebounding may be able to jump for only 30 seconds to a minute, but a week later find they are able to rebound more than ten minutes without getting tired. Space flight and bed rest reduces the number of mitochronida per cell. Rebounding or a high G force increases the number.

Enhance Your Vision with Rebound Exercise

The inability to use vision efficiently as the major sensory system to the brain can be a primary cause of learning disabilities in children as well as in adults. Treatment of these visual perception dysfunctions is called *vision therapy*. Developmental optometry, a specialty within the profession of optometry, has made effective use of rebounding for over forty years. They have found the rebounder to be a valuable tool for creating an awareness of vision as the primary guiding system for movement.

To better understand the role of rebounding in vision therapy, a brief background summary is helpful. Many parents of learning disabled children, suspecting vision problems, have consulted an optometrist for help and guidance. Symptoms, including letter and number reversal, awkward posture and handwriting, holding books very close to the eyes when reading, immaturity in physical and coordination development, and short visual attention span are reported by parents.

Often, the standard vision analysis, which measures the optical components of each eye, eye balance and efficiency of eyes to team together, provides little insight into the problem. The standard vision analysis seldom provides an adequate solution. Specialists began wondering why such obvious vision problems were not being diagnosed by routine examinations.

Research spearheaded by such notables as A. M. Skeffington, O.D., G.N. Getman, O.D., and D. B. Harmon, Ph.D., under the auspices of the Optometric Extension Program, provided some clues to the dilemma. The visual difficulties appeared to be inadequate visual perception development, usually accompanied by immaturity of other sensory systems.

We are born with the physical equipment for vision, audition, kinesthesis (movement), touch, taste, and smell. We learn to use these systems to gather information about our environment. Learning and maturing begins in infancy and continues throughout our lifetime. Taste and smell mature most quickly in infancy, followed by movement and touch, which begin maturing rapidly at six months to one year. Vision and auditory systems mature more slowly, reaching rapid development at 18 months to two years of age. The Gesell Institute of Child Development in New Haven, Connecticut has done mammoth research into human growth and development, providing much of our knowledge in this area.

In some children, sensory development of all systems appears to take place at a slower rate of speed. This may be due to inadequate environmental stimulation by parents, physical handicaps, neurological impairment, or just a slow time clock. At age five or six, when the average child is ready for school, these children are unable to use their vision and auditory systems as effective learning tools. Many of these children are still using movement and touch as primary learning modes. Unfortunately, movement and touch skills are not of much value in a classroom environment.

In rebound vision therapy, we attempt to help "Mother Nature" along in the development of the vision and vision-auditory interaction systems by creating a cellular environment where these systems will strengthen and mature at a more rapid rate. With the use of charts, we concentrate on such areas as visually-guided body movements; hand-eye coordination; visual size, space, form and directional relationships; visualization and visual memory skills. These skill areas provide the tools with which a child learns to read and do other school skills. As the skill level in these areas improves, school performance often shows a corresponding improvement.

The rebounder is used to bring about efficient visually-guided movement of the entire body. Rebounding gives magnificent feedback to what the child does thus bringing about a rapid awareness of using vision to guide movement. The rebounder is often used to bring about directional awareness, especially right and left. Confusion in this area often results in letter and word reversals.

Some developmental optometrists use the rebounder in working with athletes to develop better concentration when participating in their individual sport.

In May 1979, The National Institute of Reboundology and Health, Inc., sent a survey to everyone we could find who was involved with rebound exercise. Although we learned a lot from the returns of the survey, the answer that has influenced us more than any other was when we found that 19% of all who answered the survey registered a visual improvement through rebound exercise! This survey was taken before *The Miracles of Rebound Exercise* was made available, and before most people were aware that vision could be improved by rebounding. The Institute developed a visual re-education program which included charts, a cassette tape on how to use the charts and visual therapy techniques used while rebounding. We sold 10,000 of these vision therapy kits with a money-back guarantee, followed up with another survey, and found that a whopping 82% improved their vision!

It is an accepted fact that to achieve good health, one must have access to sound nutrition, proper exercise, pure water, and a positive mental attitude. Healthy vision not only needs all these prerequisites, but another that should be included is "correct knowledge." It is a common misconception that the eyes and maintenance of good sound vision are the responsibilities of the professional eye doctor. We expect them to store visual knowledge so that we don't have to bother about the details of the health of our own eyes. More than a dozen books have been written on visual therapy outlining the results people achieve by practicing various exercise techniques. Visual therapy is not a dream, but a reality. It works.

In preparation for eye improvement work, be ready to receive other benefits besides improved vision. It is almost impossible to improve the eyes without improving the whole body. The cells that make up the eyes are functionally the same as the cells that make up the rest of the body. Therefore, what's good for the cells of the eyes is also good for the cells of the entire body. Likewise, any healthy activity that makes the body healthier will also aid in improving vision.

The Ruth Dunlap Story

At age 44, Ruth Dunlap, of Uhrichsville, Ohio, was told by her doctor that she had multiple sclerosis. She was seeing double, could barely walk straight, and her left leg was numb.

A friend, concerned about her wellbeing, introduced her to rebound exercise. After reading chapter 12 in *The Miracles of Rebound Exercise,* she began to experiment with her vision while rebounding. She decided to go back to her old prescription lenses to see if she could adjust her vision.

Just as soon as she could see with those lenses, she switched again to an even older pair of glasses. She continued this process until she was able to use glasses prescribed for her in 1954 - over thirty years previously! Ruth is determined to continue her vision improvement until she no longer needs glasses.

At this writing, the vision therapy kit is out of print, but a book entitled *Enhance Your Vision with Rebound Exercise* is being written and will be out soon. Look for it.

Rebound Education

Vision therapists have been using small trampolines for years to help patients develop better vision. Most people believe that vision is hereditary, and therefore unquestioningly accept their visual handicaps. Visual therapists have found that vision is a learned procedure and is subject to training. Through the experience of many optometrists and educators, there is overwhelming evidence that most students do not learn to see well enough by the time they start school. The teacher, the parent, and the child all fight a losing battle when the child's ability to see is poorly developed. As children learn to visualize, they learn to look and observe. They learn to see with less time. They gain the visual ability to substitute symbols for experience. They learn simple hand and finger manipulation as a visual activity, which, when properly applied, produces a good writer, a good reader, and a good speller. Because 80% of everything we learn comes through the eye, good visual training is vital throughout the education process.

1. *Gross Motor Control* is the ability to move the body where and when one wants to.

2. *Eye-Hand Control* is the ability to direct the hand with visual clues.

3. *Eye Control* is the ability to focus the eyes and identify objects correctly.

4. *Visualization* is the ability to remember objects, clues, and symbols, memorize things, and dream of past experiences and abstract concepts.

5. *Visual-Auditory-Language* relations is the ability to read,

write, and describe what is seen or read.

6. *Organization* is the ability to interrelate all five of the above skills.

The original *Miracles* had just a few pages dedicated to rebound education. This revolutionary idea has been expanded to a complete book on the subject. Look for it under the title of *Rebound Education.* With the use of this book, parents and teachers will be able to become actively involved in the visual and educational training of their children and students in a fun and highly effective way.

On the rebounder, rhythm and timing are essential to the student's learning activities; constant and steady rhythm must become adequate in neuromuscular coordination. Because incorrect rhythm is noticed by the parent or instructor immediately, instant feedback is provided showing whether the desired response is correct.

Regardless of the participant's age, rebound exercise will help these aspects of his learning life:

1) Balance
2) Tactile and kinesthetic awareness
3) Positive body image
4) Coordination
5) Spacial awareness
6) Timing
7) Rhythm
8) Self-confidence
9) Attention span
10) Behavior
11) Problem solving and positive learning skills
12) Visualization/memory
13) Voluntary muscle action
14) Breathing habits
15) Endurance
16) Caloric burn
17) Lymphatic circulation

18) Self-esteem

Reading the original *Miracles* has brought enlightenment to teachers all over the world. They find that children who were formerly failing the first or second grade are now able to achieve A and B grades. Visual therapists are now recommending rebounding to psychiatrists and special education instructors because they see such phenomenal improvements. "Rebound exercise provides opportunities for the acquisition of basic movement control, which is essential to coordination," so states Dr. G. N. Getman, O.D. Studies before and after the publication of *The Miracles of Rebound Exercise* indicate that rebounding can provide positive experiences which influence a child's academic success. But is educational improvement limited to only the children? No. Those who wish to improve their personal skills, whether a Ph.D., a golfer, a high school student, an attorney, a mentally-slow student or an Olympic athlete, rebound education can enhance their lives. We cover rebound education in our Reboundology Seminar, and have since the beginning. But this information is so important that *everyone* needs to know. That's why the book, *Rebound Education* is a must for parents and teachers. In this book, we share with you some of the techniques other educators have found beneficial as they explore the use of this new and gratifying tool.

Rebound Exercise and The Athlete

In late 1977 during one of my lectures in Bellevue, Washington, I was explaining the theory of rebound exercise. Gideon Ariel, Ph.D., was in the audience. He has been featured in *Sports Illustrated* numerous times and featured more than once on *20/20* as one of the foremost biomechanical scientists in the nation. He has been commissioned several times to study various aspects of rebound exercise. Half-way through my presentation Ariel stood up and walked to the back of the room. This disturbed me so much that I couldn't continue. I announced a break and walked to the back of the room myself.

Seeing me come toward him, Ariel said, "Al, you have just explained why the results of one of my tests turned out so positive."

He was referring to a group of tennis players who used rebounding as a tennis teaching aid. In comparing the results to a control group, Ariel was able to conclude that a player using rebound exercise as a tennis teaching aid in practice drills can expect to improve his accuracy and efficiency more than 100% over the players who don't rebound.

George Janson, the Athletic Director of Tiffin University, dropped his golf score from 100 to the low 80s!

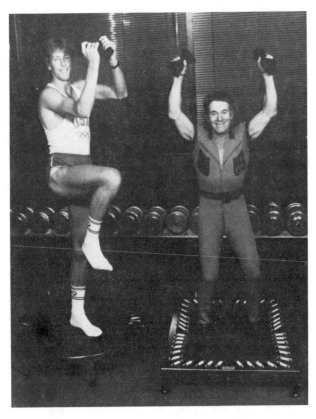

Dwight Stones with Jack LaLanne

Dwight Stones, America's high-jump record holder in 1976 set a new American high-jump record while preparing for the '84 Olympics after he had been rebounding for two years under the close supervision of Dr. Harry Sneider, the Olympic Track and Field coach at Ambassador College.

Coming Attractions:

Yes, *Rebound To A Better Athlete* is yet another book which you should look for if you are interested in improving your athletic skills.

Some of the other titles which might pique your interest include:

Executive Rebounding, Rebound Exercise and the Woman, and *Therapeutic Rebounding.*

CHAPTER 6

HISTORICALLY SPEAKING

Those of you who were involved in the rebound craze in the beginning will remember that, back in 1976, there were only two rebound devices available. *The Sundancer,* manufactured in Las Vegas, Nevada, and the *Pacer Mat* from Texas. The Sundancer was round and expensive, but well-built. The Pacer Mat was rectangular and expensive, but the seven-inch legs could not keep the participant from hitting the floor, especially since it had springs in the four legs to act as shock absorbers to reduce spring-breakage. The year 1977 ended with at least five manufacturers competing for a market that was just becoming aware of the health benefits of exercise in general, and more specifically, rebound exercise. Trampolining as an industry was down-and-out at the count of ten by then. Those who remembered how exhilarating it was to jump on a trampoline in school were having children of their own. It was a natural move for many to look to the in-house jumping-jogger, or, as the general public began to call 'em, mini-trampolines.

During the next three years, a real rebound industry began

to take shape. All the intrigue of any other aggressive industry was going on right in our own back yard, so to speak. Corporate piracy, slander, shooting down the competition, undercutting, price gouging, and mass media advertising abounded. Securing endorsements and paying off the right people to secure the right amount of leverage followed.

Multi-level marketing companies and their independent distributors began buying literature by the hundreds and even thousands. The more literature that was sold, the more people became involved, either as a seller or as a consumer.

The National Institute of Reboundology and Health, Inc., marveled at the luck of the timing. An entire industry needed what we had - rebound education. Naturally we fanned the flames. News letters were sent to everybody we knew who were involved in any way in rebounding telling them how well others were doing. One-page flyers were produced and sold in bulk. Books were published, *Rebound to Better Health, Rebounding Aerobics, Bouncerize, The Olympic Trainer*. We became a specialty-publisher and we aggressively attacked the market, expanding it and massaging it like pizza dough.

We published a list of over one hundred known United States manufacturers near the beginning of 1981. Although they were manufacturing rebound devices of all shapes and sizes (one was even made of a truck tire innertube covered with a strong fish net; (the more air in the tube, the more bounce you got out of the net stretched across the middle of the tube), most of them were back ordered by sixty days. Those were the days of rebound glory! Then it happened - almost over night.

I remember it well. Within one week, five different manufacturers called me to report that they had just secured the national contract to supply Montgomery Wards with their rebounders. At first we were elated, because naturally that meant more book sales. Then the reality of what happened began to hit us. All five manufacturers could not have secured the national contract for Wards. A few well placed telephone calls provided the real story. Five different regional offices were allowed to accept supply contracts to see which one of the five could supply the cheapest unit. It was Wards method of driving down the price. The price did drop - so did the quality of the materials used to manufacture the units. Finally, M & M Products, of Denver won the national contract for Wards simply because they underbid all other competition. Their bid was "a dollar an inch in diameter." A thirty-six inch diameter rebounder wholesaled to Wards for $36.00. A forty-inch diameter, $40.00. The lowest bid is not always the best bid, as M & M soon found out. They lost an average of $2.27 for every unit they manufactured. Soon what had been a gold mine turned into a corporate grave. Taking their cue from Wards; Pennys and Sears, other mass-merchandizers began to offer rebound exercisers.

Asian Competition

The craze caught the attention of foreign manufacturers. Soon rebounders were coming into U.S. ports by the thousands, and they were being sold for as little as $29.95 in the stores. The foreign manufacturers didn't understand anything about reboundology. All they knew was Americans, for some reason, had this crazy urge to jump up and down on a bouncy surface supported by springs attached to a frame. They knew they could beat the wholesale price by 1) further cheapening the material, and 2) cheaper construction labor.

Price War - Rebounding Has Its Ups and Downs

The foreign manufacturers stole the market with units retailing in drugstores and even some supermarkets at $19.95. Most of the U.S. manufacturers went out of business. The price war on rebounders had finally run its course.

More than a million and a half rebounders were sold in 1983. These figures were up by more than 33% over 1982, when an astounding 72 million dollars was spent by consumers on rebounders! In 1984, department stores, discount stores, sporting goods stores, and even drugstores accounted for more than 78% of all sales of rebound units. These are the rebounders which disgusted consumers pitched into the trash when the springs were sprung, or the legs broke off, or the mat split. The original dedicated U.S. manufacturers responsible for starting the industry took in only 13% of the sales volume. Why? Their actual construction costs were more than the full price of the cheap units.

The Dark Ages of Rebound Exercise

For the next eighteen months, cheap rebounders were available at almost every consumer outlet. People bought them not because they knew anything about the physical effects rebounding had on the body, but because everybody else seemed to be buying them. It was simply "the thing to do." The mass merchandizers were not buying rebound education literature because "educating the public isn't our job." Those who used to distribute literature were not making any money, so they were not buying literature. Rather than sell our literature to the distributors of the cheaper units, The National Institute of Reboundology and Health, Inc. closed its doors. To make money to support my family, I accepted an invitation from Mike Colburn, (an enthusiastic rebounder who had read *Miracles* in London and moved to Australia), to go to Australia. He assured me I would be welcome there.

Australia - The Land of the Ultimate Rebounder - The Kangaroo

Rebound exercise was just beginning to be introduced "down under". This seemed strange to me because they had kangaroos rebounding all over the outback. However, the kangaroo did become an example of rebound exercise in my lectures. "How do you think they developed those oversized, extremely powerful hind legs?" I asked.

The farther you get away from home, the more of a hero you become. I was welcomed by everybody as the next health expert on the horizon, or beyond the horizon, I guess.

National television interviews and newspaper interviews were expected of me. My every waking moment was filled giving exercise advice to the friendly people of Australia. My Reboundology Seminars were filled to capacity. It was as if they could not get enough of the information I had tried so hard to make available in the United States. I was beginning to think I had died and gone to Rebound Heaven.

One day, just before I was about to go on television, Mike slipped me a note that said a Mr. Peter Daetweiler of Hong Kong would like to speak to me. Being extremely busy and not knowing anybody in Hong Kong, I ignored the message. However, the third time I received the same note thrust into my palm in two days, I decided that Peter what-ever-his-name-was deserved a return call.

The fraction of a second delay in the over-seas telephone conversation didn't hide the effervescent personality of Mr. Daetweiler, who informed me that he had been trying to locate me for the last three weeks. He convinced me, after just a few minutes of conversation, that I should "drop in on him since I was in his neighborhood." (Some people's neighborhoods are bigger than others.) I rearranged my homeward bound flight to spend three days in Hong kong to meet the body of this very pleasing and persuasive personality.

Hong Kong Rebounds

"Paging arriving passenger Mr. Albert Carter of flight 005, United Airlines. Please meet your party at Customs Exit." It was a good thing Mr. Daetweiler sent an automobile to pick me up. I had no idea where I was going in this country that was so proud of its own heritage. As I left customs, I saw a small hand-printed sign on a stick two feet above the heads of the pedestrians. "Mr. Albert Carter." All of the "Rs" were backwards, but it was close enough. Instead of one person to pick me up, there were three, two men and one woman. All were dressed in the same dark-blue suits and white silk shirts. My luggage was immediately (but carefully) fitted into the open trunk of a late model Mercedes Benz. I was tucked away into the air-conditioned back seat. Brief introductions were shared and away we went through the bustling streets of Hong Kong. Arriving at the Holiday Inn in Kaloon, we stopped at the front desk only long enough for me to register on our way up to the fourteenth floor, and a very welcome and luxurious room.

"Please enjoy your stay. You are free this evening." explained Charlie Lo. "Mr. Daetweiler will see you at 8:30 in the morning. Your meals are on the house." The doors closed and I was alone in a strange world filled with funny (to me) sounding people waiting for morning.

At first impression, the man was exactly like his voice; enthusiastic, charisimatic. What the voice and the body did not tell me, his private secretary did while I waited in his outer office until precisely 8:30 am. Mr. Daetweiler was the Czar of Holiday Inn in the South Pacific Theatre. He was the chief

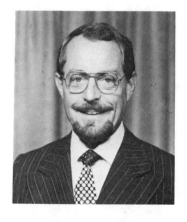

Peter Daetweiler

administrator over twenty-seven luxury hotels strategically placed in Singapore, Taiwan, Bangkok, Japan, the Philippines, New Zealand, and anywhere else Holiday Inn could serve the tourist trade. His rigorous regimen was timed to the quarter of a minute. He kept three secretaries busy. His orders were sharp, snapped out like a whip, and his decisions were quick and final. His flowing face and trim body attested that his regimented lifestyle did not stop with his business.

"Good morning, Mr. Carter. Your accommodations are to your liking?" He asked sincerely, but I believe he was also checking on his subjects.

"Beyond expectations," I replied honestly.

"I read your book eleven months ago, (if he had read it eleven months and two days ago, he would have said eleven months and two days) when I was introduced to rebound exercise. I had been running an hour three days a week for over two years when I developed pain in my left knee. It became necessary to have my doctor shoot it with coritsone just about every week to control the pain and swelling just so I could continue to run. Then one of my friends asked me if I knew anything about rebounding, and she presented me with your book. I read your book and she sold me a rebounder and I've been rebounding every day since then without pain. The knee is as good as new."

"I'm glad to hear the book was beneficial to you," I said diplomatically.

"Beneficial! It changed my life! I thought I was getting older, but now I'm just getting better!"

"I truly appreciate your enthusiastic testimonial, Mr. Daetweiler..."

"Peter," he interrupted.

"Thank you, Peter, but I am sure you invited me to Hong Kong for something more than praising my book."

"Lynn Chee, bring me the South China Morning Post," he said into his intercom. At almost the same moment, Miss Chee opened the door with a copy of the morning newspaper.

"You can stop this," he said with certainty in his voice as he turned the front page to me.

Half way down the page the headlines read:

"FIRE AND POLICE STRIKE SCHEDULED,
NEGOTIATIONS BROKEN OFF"

"You want me to stop a strike??' I asked.

"You are probably the only one in the world who can do it right now."

"I know nothing of mediation." I exclaimed.

"They don't need a mediator. They need a problem solved. Once the problem is solved, mediation isn't necessary."

"What problem can I solve, Peter?"

"Their problem. The Hong Kong Government has demanded that all police and fire personnel carry on a personal exercise program to keep in top emergency physical fitness."

"That's great!" I exclaimed. "I wish the policemen and firemen in the United States had the same requirement. Don't they want to?"

"Yes. They are willing to keep in shape. The policemen and firemen want to do it on company time. . ."

"And the government wants them to do it on their own time." I finished.

"Exactly. There are legitimate arguments on both sides. You are talking valuable time and money either way. There are seven thousand firemen and twenty-eight thousand police officers. That is why neither side is willing to budge."

"Wow. That isn't just a small army."

"Al, you haven't seen much of Hong Kong, but I am sure it is confusing to you."

"You got that right."

"For the number of people who live here, it runs pretty smoothly only because of the tight control the police and fire departments have on the unsavory elements," he explained. "There is no way you could imagine what this place would be like without police protection."

"Peter, what makes you think I could have any effect on the outcome of the impending strike?"

"Because their method of exercise is jogging. Here, read this." He pointed to a part of the paper and then proceeded to read aloud: " 'As high as twenty percent of the police officers are limping while walking their patrol'. . . Al, I was one of those because I used to run with them! You can help them"

"How can I be sure they will listen to me?"

"You leave that to me. That's the easy part. We'll start by your being my guest tonight at a political dinner. Both the Fire Chief and the Chief of Police will be sitting at my table. Tomorrow we will seek an audience with Hilton Cheong-Leen, Chairman of the Urban Council. Now, if you will excuse me, I need to be about my inspection tour of the hotel. My driver will pick you up at 6:30 pm.

I was ushered out as quickly as I came in and left with the rest of the day to wander around the streets of Hong Kong. I wondered what it was going to be like ten days from now without the police protection. It was a good thing I was staying for only three days.

Early the next morning, the secretary ushered us into the inner office of the Chairman of the Urban Council. Impeccably dressed in a western-style, tailored suit, Hilton Cheong-Leen stood and greeted us.

"Mr. Carter. It is an honor to meet you. Peter has been telling me about you and your work. I do hope that you have just one of the miracles you write about in your book for us."

"It is indeed an honor meeting with you this morning. From what Mr. Daetweiler was telling me, the miracle you speak of is a real possibility," I answered.

"You realize we have less than ten days to cut the lighted fuse of a bomb that could devastate the economy of the entire Hong Kong Commonwealth. If the police go out on strike, there's no telling when we will get them back. I don't think Hong Kong could stand a weekend without police protection, let alone the uncertainties of an extended strike."

"Mr. Daetweiler tells me that the accepted method of exercise is jogging."

"Three days a week, with weight-lifting on the off days." he clarified.

"I also understand that this exercise is supposed to be done on their own time."

"That's right. By the time they change clothes, go to an accepted running track, stretch and warm up, run, cool down, change clothes and shower, their jogging exercise takes them away from their post for two hours. It's the same way when they lift weights."

"If I can show you how to cut their exercise time to just ten minutes three times per day, and if your police and firemen can perform the necessary aerobic and strength exercises to the required standards without leaving their posts, would you then allow them to exercise on company time.?"

"That would be a miracle, and yes we could allow them to exercise on company time as long as they are within reach of a telephone or radio for the emergencies."

"Then Mr. Cheon-Leen, have I got a deal for you." With that, I began to explain how rebounding is a cellular exercise, providing the G force resistance necessary to cause all of the cells to become stronger. I demonstrated rebound running to show how easy it is to achieve aerobic endurance without having to spend time stretching, because the running surface was forgiving. I was into the middle of the strength bounce demonstrating the effect of a two G force when he stopped me.

"Rather than having you go through this demonstration again," he said, " let me call in the two chiefs."

Peter knew the way the Chairman worked. What we didn't tell Mr. Cheon-Leen is that we had already met with the chiefs informally over a fantastic oriental dinner. Our demonstration late last night ended with Mr. Daetweiler warning them to stay close to their office and to expect a call from the chairman.

At the end of the meeting, it was decided that the Chief of Police and the Fire Chief would give in to the demands of the two unions. The union members would be able to exercise on the job, but they had to exercise in a revolutionary new way just recently discovered and researched by the government. If they bought rebounding, a crippling strike would be averted.

"We had better order some rebounders for testing," Hilton Cheon-Leen suggested.

"We have a dozen on the way." Peter lied, winking at me. They will be here within a week."

That's how you sell a foreign government on rebound exercise. It took less time and effort than a simple home demonstration. The numbers were different. We just sold 20,000 rebounders of the one that held up the best after being tested. That day, I made six phone calls to six rebound manufacturing plants in the United States, asking them to send two units to me in Hong Kong ASAP, in care of the Holiday Inn in Kowloon. That day, Hong Kong displaced the North Pole as being the top of the world, for me, anyway. My next phone call was to Bonnie to let her know that I was going to

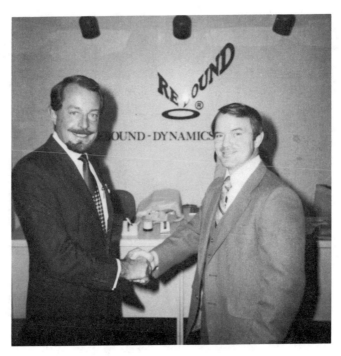

extend my stay in Hong Kong to three months instead of the three days.

The first two weeks were great! Strike averted. International hero. Newspaper and television interviews. A Public Relations staff was assigned to me, and I was personally invited to stay with one of the American Consulates while I was there. I set up an office in Kowloon with my new partner, Peter Daetweiler, under the name of Rebound Dynamics, Ltd. and we shook on it.

The Development of the Ideal High-Quality Rebounder

It was in the third week that Mr. Cheon-Leen called me personally and reported that all twelve of the rebounders had failed the test of multiple personnel usage. He requested my immediate attendance that afternoon in his office. I was there fifteen minutes later, (something you can't accomplish in the

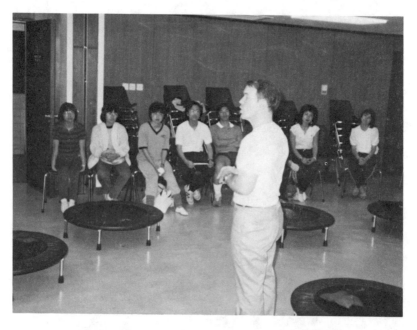

Some of Frank Drake's staff of teachers.

United States.)

"We are committed to rebound exercise," he announced starting the meeting the minute I arrived. "But the construction needs to be improved. Mr. Carter is the expert on the concept, but it is your responsibility to make sure that the equipment is the best money can buy," he said to three other men in the meeting. "Mr. Carter, these three engineers are assigned to you until you can present us with a rebound device that will hold up under the daily usage of an active police patrol. You have only two weeks to develop the working model, and another two weeks for full production of twenty thousand units. In the meantime, I have assigned Frank Drake of the Sports and Recreation Department to help you develop a rebound teaching system they can use afer you leave. You should plan your time to work in the mornings with the engineers, and in the afternoons with Mr. Drake's staff of teachers. Remember, we have accepted the rebound concept. It is impossible for you to fail. We cannot allow it. We would never live it down."

At that moment, Hong Kong slipped from the top of the world to the bottom and I felt the whole weight of the world on my shoulders. The glory was gone. Only work and stress was ahead.

Actually the rebounder came together faster than I expected. The engineers were sharp. We dissected the available devices and started from the very beginning.

Question: "Why is it round? Why not square?"

Answer: A circle is the strongest geometric structure in a single plane.

Question: Why is the bouncing surface eight inches off the ground? Why not seven or nine?

Answer: It has to be high enough so that a three hundred pound participant cannot hit the floor while bouncing as high as possible, yet low enough so that a six-foot, two-inch person does not hurt himself by hitting a standard ceiling. In Hong Kong, the standard ceilings are lower, but then so are the people, so the eight-inch height was the best for both Hong Kong and the United States.

Question: Can we use a cheaper material for the bouncing surface. For example, nylon, canvas or plastic?

Answer: All three fabrics stretch. Once they stretch out-of-shape, the rebounder has lost its resiliency. Permatron is more expensive, but it's the only fabric that doesn't stretch. It is also more durable than the other fabrics and outlasts them three to one.

Question: What is the best grade of wire to make the springs?

Answer: .6 of 1% carbon steel stretches, .72 of 1% carbon steel wire is too brittle. We decided to go with the number eighty carbon steel. Although it's more expensive, .8 of 1% carbon steel springs maintain their resiliency much longer.

Question: Is there a better way to connect the spring to the frame so that the spring doesn't wear through the metal? All twelve sample units connected their springs by drilling a hole in the frame and connecting the end of the spring in the hole. In just two weeks, the springs had worn through the frame in thirty-six different places. At that rate, we would have to replace the frames every ninety days.

Answer: The engineers came up with a bolt through the frame. They pointed out that the bolt was five times as thick as the frame and that it would be more economical to replace the bolts

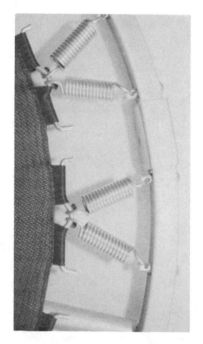

"ProBounder 2000"

than the entire frame. With nothing wearing on the frame, the frame should last forever.

Question: Space is of a premium in Hong Kong. Is there a way to store the rebounder when not in use?

Answer: The solid circle frame can be cut in half and hinged. To keep it from folding while in use, the hinges have to be off-center and upside-down. The off-center hinges would require a special effort to fold the unit. Since the unit folds upside-down, the only time it could possibly be folded is when somebody purposely turned it upside-down to fold it.

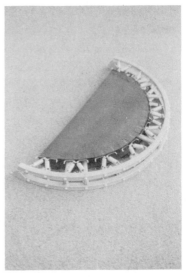

"ProBounder 2000"

Question: Legs that screw on can potentially strip the threads or lose a leg when unattached. Is there a quick secure way of folding the legs to eliminate loss potential or malfunction because of stripped threads?

Answer: The engineers developed a unique leg that is attached with a spring inside the leg. It provides positive tension while the unit is in use, but can be folded with a one inch outward pull. The addition of the folding legs and the folding frame makes it possible to fold or unfold the unit in less than

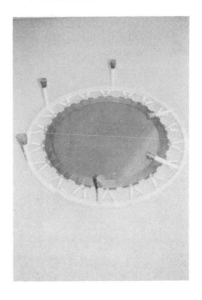

"ProBounder 2000"

fifteen seconds. The folded unit is small enough to fit in the trunk of a car, the back of a closet, under the bed, and the overhead luggage bin in most airplanes. It is also small enough to be shipped by United Parcel Service. That reduces the shipping cost in the United States to only one fourth the trucking rates.

There are a dozen other improvements the engineers made over the existing rebound devices. When we were satisfied, we contracted with a company to produce them. In exchange for my services in Hong Kong, I received the authority to produce this perfected unit and market it throughout the rest of the world.

When I first submitted the working model to several factories in the United States, I was surprised to find that their best production cost at that time would be too exorbitant. I was forced to turn to Taiwan to produce the unit so I could keep the cost as low as possible while still maintaining a high standard of quality.

Fortunately since then, the U.S. has jumped on the bandwagon of production and I have gladly contracted with one factory to produce a unit not only equal but superior to any rebounder unit on the market. I an so pleased with this new unit I have renamed it **ProBounder 2000.**

As other health officials of other departments became aware of rebounding, I became more than just a little busy. Hong Kong is a socialistic government. For the most part, health maintenance and medical attention are free to the citizenry because the government pays socialistic medicine. Therefore, personal health is a responsibility of the government. The healthier it can keep its population, the more money it saves on overall medical costs. Nursing homes for the aged began to call for me. We made Reboundology Seminars available to physiologists and physical therapists. Dr. Charles Low, Administrator of the Physical Education Department of the University of Hong Kong, saw to it that at least fifty percent of

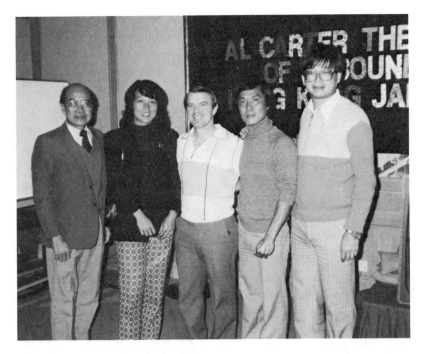

Dr. Charles Low (left) and author in the middle with three members of his University of Hong Kong staff.

his staff became Certified Reboundologists. The girls' tennis team of the Hong Kong University (pictured on page 84) developed a choreographed chorus line using rebound exercise to develop their physical capabilities for playing tennis. This bouncy musical presentation was presented to over four thousand of the tennis-playing public one evening just before John MacEnroe played an exhibition match with one of Hong Kong's greatest tennis players.

Needless to say, rebounding swept Hong Kong in just a few short months. Everybody who was anybody was doing it. Political figures wanted their picture taken with me to let the rest of the people know they were part of the "in-the-know-crowd."

The civic organizsations, Kiwanis, Rotary and Lions Clubs, invited me to speak to their members. The meetings were

picture of girls' tennis team

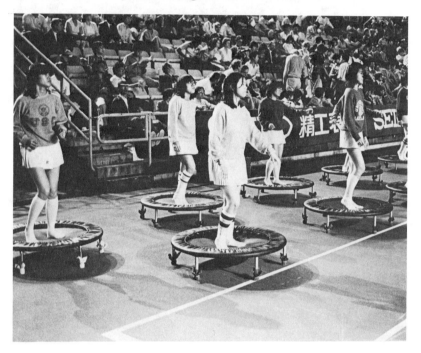

beyond successful educational presentations. Of the one hundred ten Rotarians who were present at the Hong Kong Rotary Club when I was the guest speaker, forty-nine

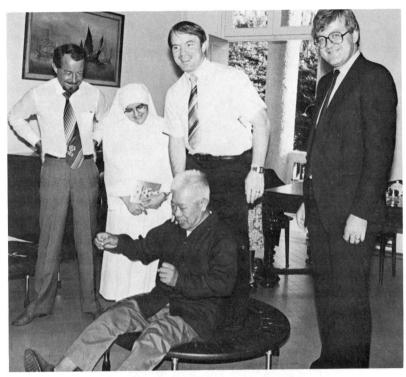

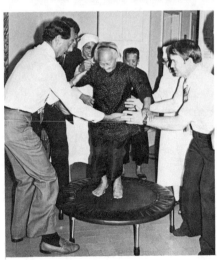

Rebounding is for the elderly: Those who can't walk and those who can.

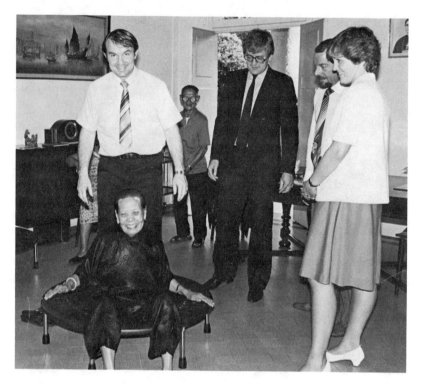

purchased units.

The prestigious Hong Kong Health Club purchased a supply for the use of their members.

Business people from other countries visiting Hong Kong on other business became enamoured with this latest business opportunity. I remember one of my Reboundology Seminars included representatives from Hong Kong, Taiwan, Singapore, New Zealand, Australia, Philippines, Bangkok, Switzerland, Israel, England, Japan, The United States, and Canada. Each contingent wanted to take the rebound message back to their own countries. We began to sell rebounders by forty-foot containers (each container contains over one thousand rebounders) to these international entrepreneurs.

What more could a person ask of one life than to be accepted as the World's foremost authority on any subject, let alone rebound exercise, the most efficient effective form of

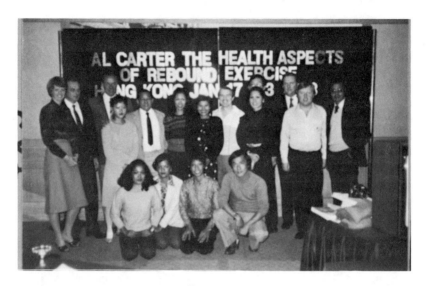

exercise yet devised by man?

The Hong Kong Sports and Recreation Department put together a twelve person task force dedicated to understanding and disseminating the principles of rebounding in Cantonese, Mandarin, and other local dialects. All were bilingual. I spoke in English, and they wrote their teaching manuals in their various languages. It became necessary for me to not only understand the principles behind rebounding, but also to be able to explain in a logical sequence the exercise movements that could be accomplished on the rebounder, and to teach how each movement directly affected the various parts of the body. It wasn't long before we began to recognize a definite relationship between the exercises. As we recognized patterns, we began to classify movements.

Although they thought I had this all worked out in advance, I was amazed at the logical way in which all possible movements could be classified into four major bounces, plus two other classifications. The bounces became: *Health Bounces; Aerobic Bounces; Strength Bounces;* and *Sitting Bounces.* The other classification was: *Turns* and *Kicks.* All other rebound activities can be sub-classified under one of these headings.

CHAPTER 7

REBOUND EXERCISE CATEGORIZED

In this chapter, because a picture is worth a thousand words, we're going to *show* you exactly how to rebound to best advantage, as well as describe the moves in the text. I promise you that rebounding is the best, most efficient exercise ever devised by man. What's more, it's actually fun! But first, there's someone I want you to meet.

She's Not A Model...

Sylvia Ortiz, shown demonstrating some advanced moves on ProBounder 2000 on many of the following pages, is not a model. She just looks like one. It's her healthy lifestyle that gives her the svelte figure, fresh complexion, and that irresistible smile.

During her teen years in high school, this petite 5'3" dynamo confesses she was seventy-eight pounds overweight. In spite of her undeniably pretty face and luxurious mane of hair, the excess weight she was carrying around back then left her feeling self-conscious and depressed. She hated looking in her mirror.

To make matters worse, Sylvia developed a serious

condition that the doctors had a hard time diagnosing. It was finally determined that her gall bladder wasn't functioning as it should, a direct result of the junk-food diet that had led to her obesity. At age 17, Sylvia underwent surgery to remove her gall bladder. The surgery was doubly complicated because of the excess fat that surrounded the organ. She carries a six inch long vertical scar (she calls it her 'zipper') running from her breast bone down to her navel.

As she lay in bed recovering from this major operation, Sylvia took stock of herself. The doctors had already explained that it would be necessary for her to follow a healthy diet for life. Without her gall bladder, certain foods would be impossible for her body to process. This fact provided the impetus she needed to slim down.

She had tried to lose weight many times before. Her intentions were always good, but she was fighting a losing battle. Her bad eating habits, which stimulated powerful cravings for the wrong foods, played havoc with her willpower. A war raged within her body. It wasn't until she took a behavior modification course, coupled with a crash-course on nutrition, that she was able to establish good eating habits. She won only the small battles at first, but eventually was completely victorious. She ate a lot of fresh fruit and followed the diet her doctor prescribed carefully.

As soon as she was up and around, Sylvia began the regimen of walks her doctor had ordered. Her progress was slow and she puffed as she made her way around the block. Until this time of her life, she had never exercised. She hated it, but perservered. So gradually that she was not at first aware of it, she found she had picked up the pace. Soon, instead of dreading it as an ordeal to suffer through, she was looking forward to her walks. The pounds began dropping off and she began to get excited.

After a few months, her walking regimen turned to jogging. When she reached her 'fighting' weight of 108 pounds, jogging wasn't enough any more. Sylvia began to run in earnest. She ran for the sheer joy of it. As she slimmed down, her body tightened up and her muscles became softly defined. The obese teenager that had been the object of ridicule was no more. The personality and sparkle and exuberance that marks her today came forth. She laughed a lot and flashed her Latin eyes and the boys came running. By the time twelve months had passed, Sylvia was transformed into one of the most popular girls in school. She had come into her own and she reveled in it.

If you think that's the 'happy ending' to Sylvia's story, you're wrong. When she was 24 years old, she married and soon a child was born. Now in near-perfect health, Sylvia bounced back from the birth quickly. At this point in time, she was running fifty miles per week and felt wonderfully alive. But her dark days were not yet behind her.

With her six month-old baby son held in her arms, Sylvia stumbled coming down a long flight of hard wood steps. The young mother instinctively protected her infant. Without conscious thought, she used her own body to shield her child. Because she refused to break her fall with her hands, the accident had severe consequences for Sylvia. The baby was shaken up a bit and slightly bruised.

But Sylvia's tailbone was broken. Yet again, she faced major surgery and the long road back to health. But this time she had an edge. Her superb physical condition stood her in good stead. She was bedridden off and on for a year. Impatient as she was to get going again out on the track, there was absolutely nothing she could do. She knew her hard won physical gains were deteriorating and she could feel her muscles begin to atrophy and slacken as the long months went by.

Sylvia explains, "I felt useless. Exercise is the very soul of my existence! I fell into a depression. Not being able to exercise was unbearable to me. To compound my frustration, I became aware that the pounds were packing back on because of my inactivity. This panicked me. After eight years of healthy eating and a hard-driving jogging regimen, I was terrified that the seventy pounds I had lost were edging back on."

Finally the day came when her doctors said she could begin an exercise regimen again. But running was forbidden. Too much shock to the musculoskeletal system, they explained. Sylvia was discouraged at the thought that running might cause further damage to her now weakened back, but determined that she would find an adequate substitute for her runs in the park. It was then that she discovered rebounding.

Sylvia says, "Even though my doctor said I could begin limited exercise, I was still suffering intense pain. I wasn't sure he was right and consequently sought medical attention from various physicians and other health professionals. Among these was a chiropractor who was an advocate of rebound aerobics. He was well ahead of the times." (Note: Today, Dr. Karl Parker, Executive V.P. of Parker Chiropractic Resource Foundation, endorses rebounding and offers ProBounder 2000 and my books in his catalog.)

Sylvia continues, "Dr. Jeff Gamble encouraged me to try the rebounder for exercise. I was very skeptical. The last thing I wanted was to be bedridden again, and I was sure I would get killed using that contraption. But my desire to exercise was stronger than my fear. I gave rebounding a chance. To my delight, aerobic exercise on the rebounder was easy to master. Best of all, it didn't hurt my back!"

Because the Permatron pad absorbs up to 6/8ths of the shock to the system, rebounding was ideal for Sylvia. Sylvia bought her first rebounder and began slowly building up the strength she had lost. Sooner than she had dared hope, her body became a finely-tuned instrument once again. She took note that her cardiovascular and respiratory functions were even better than when she was running fifty miles every week. A comparison with the data she had compiled on herself in her running days confirmed it.

Sylvia says happily, "My back got stronger and stronger every day. Moreover, in just three months of rebounding, I lost fifteen pounds and I no longer needed the doctors." Sylvia concluded that rebounding was not only an adequate substitute for running, it was actually better.

She was also pleased to find that rebounding was doing some subtle body shaping that she hadn't expected. Although she had been well satisfied with her body measurements before, she found her waist, hips, and thighs slimming down still further, while her upper body measurement increased slightly. This was an unexpected bonus. Sylvia was delighted.

Although the scientific backup for the 'miracles' Sylvia experienced was still in research and would not be published until 1988 when this book, *The New Miracles of Rebound Exercise,* was released, the effects were undeniable.

Before her accident, Sylvia had been employed as a medical assistant and physical therapist. Her background in the field helped her develop a safe and very effective rebounding program for herself. Realizing the dramatic effects rebounding had given her so quickly, she approached the owners of an exercise studio and pitched the idea of installing rebounders. To her great disappointment, they weren't interested.

But Sylvia was determined. She knew she was on to the best thing in exercising. She began giving personal rebound workouts in private homes and businesses. Just as she knew they would, her clients got spectacular results. As word-of-mouth 'advertising' by very satisfied customers escalated, this sideline business became very successful. Soon she had more clients than she could effectively handle. Her effervescent personality made her very popular and she was coaxed into producing a video entitled *Stay Fit Rebounding.* It was (and is) a hit. Sylvia's video has graced the pages of leading magazines, including *Shape, New Body, Self,* and *American Fitness.*

Even after she left her regular job and devoted full time to her rebounding students, there just weren't enough hours in the day to teach rebounding to everyone who flocked to her side. The time had come. After scraping together all the money she could on her own, she found additional financing and opened her own studio, *Fit For You* in Hacienda Heights, California in 1984. Needless to say, Sylvia installed 30 ProBounder 2000s and featured rebounding. *Fit For You* was an immediate success.

At this point in time, I didn't know Sylvia Ortiz from Adam. Still, sooner or later, everyone interested in rebounding finds me. Although we had spoken a few times over the telephone, we had never met. I was aware Sylvia was a big fan of rebounding and the owner of a highly successful aerobic rebounding studio. She had expressed interest in attending one of my Rebound Seminars, but the timing was always wrong somehow. Then everything came right.

I was in California anyway and decided to check out her *Fit For You* studio. I drove out to Hacienda Heights and met this dynamite little gal for the first time. To say I was impressed is an understatement.

Sylvia runs the business operation of her studio single-handed. Although she has four instructors she had personally trained assisting her, she herself still gives classes in aerobic rebounding. She teachs therapeutic rebounding for physically-disabled and handicapped clients, both to individual patients and the chiropractors themselves. She is board certified by the AFAA (Aerobics & Fitness Association of America). Sylvia is the only qualified rebound instructor in the program and gladly travels nationwide wherever she is needed to fulfill this obligation. She is also a Provider for AFAA and conducts Rebound-Aerobics Certification courses.

I wasted no time in putting Sylvia through her paces and she is now a Certified Reboundologist. It was easy. Truth to tell, she had been a Reboundologist for years. All she lacked was my name on the certification to confirm it. I wonder now why we never met before. With my ten years of clinical research on the medical benefits of rebounding, and Sylvia's five years of personal and studio experience, the combination is a natural.

Now that we have joined the yin (female) and yang (male) forces together, so to speak, we have each gained strength and power lacking before. When Sylvia works a Seminar with me, the audience now is able to see both sides of the complete picture for the first time. We are currently collaborating on a comprehensive manual for the continuing education of Certified Reboundologists. Sylvia also gives hands-on (or should that be 'feet-on'?) Rebound Workshops to keep our Certified Reboundologists up-to-date.

You will be hearing more from and about Sylvia as time goes by. Her input has been invaluable. This partnership is still in its infancy, but our dedication to rebounding and *The Healthy Cell Concept* (see Chapter 11) is equally strong.

Let's get started.

The Health Bounce

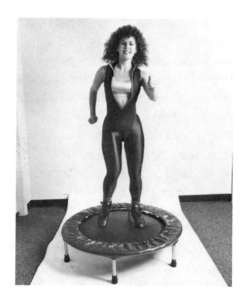

In the center of the ProBounder 2000, move up and down by using your toes and your calf muscles. Your toes will not leave the mat surface.

The Health Bounce is a good warm-up exercise. It is also good for relieving tension and improving lymphatic, or body fluid circulation. It is also used by many physiotherapists to help patients in rehabilitation. When a patient gets out of bed, exercise is vitally important, but even walking is too strenuous. Place a ProBounder 2000 next to the wall so that the patient can maintain balance by touching the wall while he does the health bounce. the health bounce stimulates the vistibular (inner ear) system, the antigravity muscles, the propreocepters (nerves) in the joints, ligaments and muscles, creating a much keener sense of balance. It is also used by vision therapists as a vision improvement exercise.

Aerobic Bounces

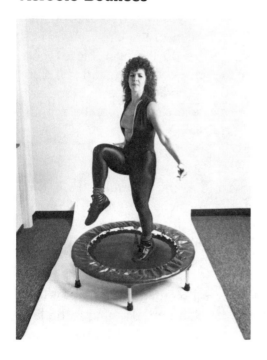

In the center of the ProBounder 2000, start a walking, jogging, or running motion in place. This can be done by leaning backward slightly and lifting your knees one at a time in front of you, or leaning forward slightly and kicking your feet out behind you. It is not necessary to wait for the rebounder to bounce your leg up. Move at your own speed.

For the purposes of classification, any activity on the ProBounder 2000 using one foot at a time would be an aerobic bounce, although all activities provide some aerobic benefits. Most of these movements are self explanatory, but we will explain them anyway as we list them.

Rebound Walk

In the center of the ProBounder 2000, begin a walking in place motion. It is best to lean back from the hips slightly and pick your feet up in front of you one at a time and replace it in the same position. Move your arms in the opposite direction. As the left foot comes up froward, the right arm moves up and forward also. The muscular movement of the large muscles of your body (arms and legs) will use up the available oxygen inside the body creating an oxygen debt. Your heart will start beating faster and you will soon be breathing deeper. You are now participating in an aerobic exercise. If your balance is questionable, put your hand on a wall.

Rebound Jog

The movements are the same as the *Rebound Walk*, only faster. However, this time it is not necessary to wait for one foot to land on the rebound mat before lifting the other. The objective is greater aerobic stimulation than the rebound walk. This can also be done by leaning slightly forward and kicking your feet out behind you. We distinguish the two by calling one the *Back Rebound Jog,* and the other the *Front Rebound Jog.* One of the benefits of the Rebound Jogging is the lack of jarring on the skeletal system.

Rebound Running

This activity is challenging to your cardiovascular system. It utilizes the same body movements as Rebound Jogging, but at a much faster pace. Don't forget to move your arms the opposite direction you move your legs, and don't wait for the mat to bounce you. Run at your own pace. This exercise is used by some of the best athletes in the world to prepare for their own athletic activity, when shinsplints, ankle problems, knee injuries or lower back pains are not only a nuisance, but could mean the difference between winning and losing, or even competing.

Rebound Sprint.

This is accomplished by moving your body the same as you would while Rebound Running, only as fast as you can. This exercise is usually short in duration because it uses up the available oxygen faster than the heart and lungs can replace the supply with fresh. It challenges the body into functioning anaerobically for short periods of time.

Elbow-Knee Crossover

This is a challenging activity for athletes. While Rebound Jogging or Running touch your left elbow with your right knee in front of you, then your right elbow with your left knee. A dozen or so ought to let you know the effectiveness and value.

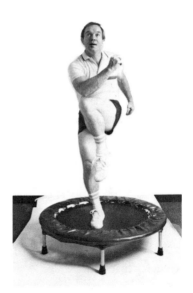

Front High Kick

In the center of the ProBounder 2000, while landing on the left foot while leaning backwards, kick the right straight out in front as high as you can, then kick the left foot out the same way while landing on the right. Swing your arms the opposite direction of your leg movement.

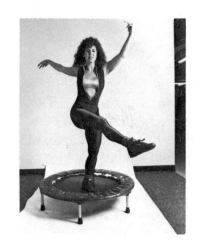

Back High Kick

Lean forward while kicking backward one foot at a time.

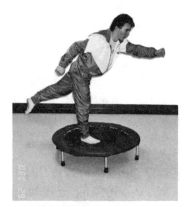

Side High Kick

Lean toward the opposite side of your kicking leg, each time you land, lean the opposite direction. This creates a sideways rocking motion.

As you become experienced in rebounding, try moving smoothly from one aerobic move to another.

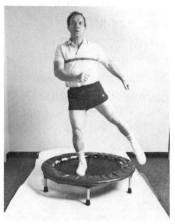

Strength Bounces

In the middle of the ProBounder 2000, bounce so that both feet leave the mat at the same time. This can be accomplished in several ways. Rhythmically shove your toes into the mat. Rhythmically bend and straighten your knees shoving your feet into the mat. Swing your arms upward in rhythm. Or, a combination of any or all will accomplish the same thing.

This is called the Strength Bounce because the vertical loading of acceleration, deceleration and gravity creates an increase in the G force to which each cell of the body has to adjust. The higher the bounce, the greater the G force.

Another benefit of the Health Bounce is the fact that your body is in free flight if only for a moment. That moment allows you to change your body and foot positions so that you are able to create an entire dance routine or aerobic workout, thus reducing the potential for boredom

Low Strength Bounce

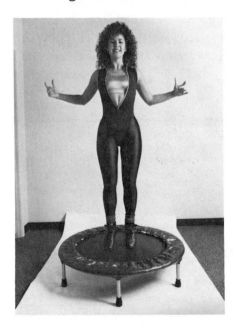

Jump so that your feet just barely leave the mat. This creates a G force anywhere from 1.1 Gs to 1.5 Gs. Touch your stomach or shoulder muscles with your finger tips. Notice that they tighten each time your land. Notice also that your can easily turn your whole body to the left or to the right with greater mobility. It is also important to learn to stay in the middle of the ProBounder 2000. Because it is safer, you are developing a greater sense of balance, and the springs will last longer.

I guess I could have introduce the *Medium Strength Bounce* here, because that's the one your will use most of the time. But what can I say about the Medium Strength Bounce, other than it's higher than the low, and lower than the High? I decided to skip that one.

High-Strength Bounce

Using the upward swing of your arms, the sudden extending of your knees, and the downward thrusting of your toes all at once to gain as much altitude as possible. This is the exercise Dr. Ward Dean of the United States Air Force measured to establish the fact that an athlete in excellent condition can develop as much as 3.24 Gs. Because the normal body can withstand as much as ten Gs with no ill effects, it has been determined scientifically that rebounding is a safe exercise for most individuals.

Shuffle Bounce

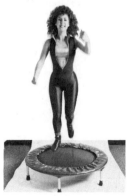

Land with one foot slightly in front of the other, and reverse on the next bounce. This will give the toes and the calves a rest because you will be landing on the heel of your forward foot instead of the toes all the time. Your legs will not tire easily, which gives the rest of your body a better work out because you won't have to stop when your legs become "too tired too soon." As soon as you have the Shuffle step mastered, you're ready to move right into the turns.

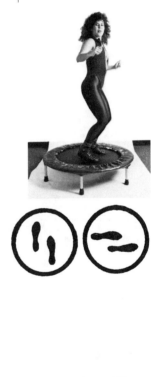

Ninety Degree Left (Right) Bounce

From the Shuffle Step with the left (right) foot back, bounce, turning to the left (right) so that you land with your left (right) foot forward and are facing 90° to the left (right). Did you get that one? or two? If you did, then you're ready for the one-eighties.

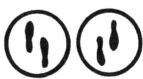

One Hundred Eighty Degree Right (Left) Bounce.

We are going to use the Shuffle Step again. With the right (left) foot back, bounce, turning 180 degrees to the right (left) so that you land facing the opposite direction with your right (left) foot forward. Now that wasn't hard was it? A bit scary, but not hard.

Three Hundred Sixty Degree Bounce

This one is both hard and scary. Don't try it until you have mastered your 180s. The approach is the same Shuffle Bounce. The direction is determined by the back foot. You land the way you left the ProBounder 2000.

Needless to say, all of the turns are terrific for the development of balance, coordination, rhythm, timing, dexterity and kinesthetic awareness.

Twist Bounce

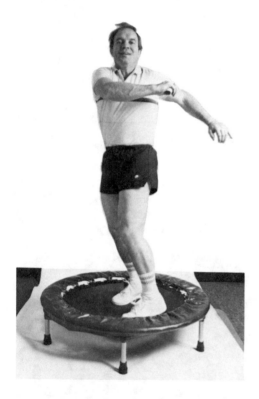

In the middle of the rebounder, bounce so that the hips and legs turn to the left and the chest and shoulders turn to the right. On the next bounce reverse it.

Slalom Bounce

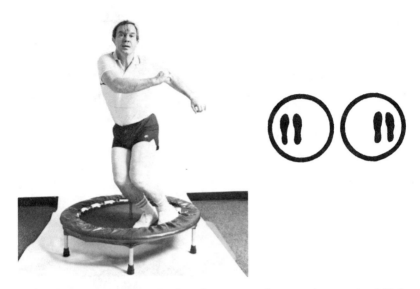

A preparatory exercise for skiing - and any other sport. With your feet positioned parallel and to the right of the center of the mat, bounce and land so that your feet are parallel and to the left of the center of the mat. Your knees and hips should absorb all of the upward movement so that your torso is virtually motionless and facing straight ahead. It is not as easy as it looks, but then, neither is skiing.

Wait! We're not finished. There's a few more movements to add a little excitement and youth to your life.

Tuck Bounce.
Using the High Strength Bounce, pull your knees up to your chest with your hands on you shins. Be sure to straighten out before landing.

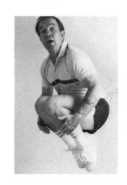

Pike Bounce

Using the High Strength Bounce again, keep the knees straight, bend sharply at the hips and touch your toes at the top of the bounce. Straighten out to vertical before you come down.

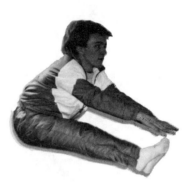

Splits Bounce

Do the splits at the top of the High Strength Bounce.

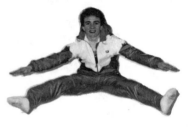

Stag Bounce

Do a stag at the top of the High Strength Bounce. If you don't know what a stag is, forget it.

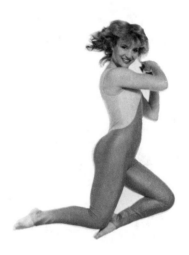

The Sitting Bounces

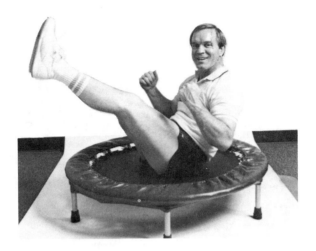

If you have been trying these exercises while I've been describing them to you, you probably need a rest. Go ahead. Sit down on the ProBounder 2000, lean back and put your hands behind you on the frame. This is an excellent position to watch television. I'm serious. When a commercial or a boring sequence happens, don't waste time, rebound. When an exciting chase scene occurs, participate by rebounding. You'll be surprised how much exercise you get if your only rebound during the commercial breaks of a movie.

Because rebounding is a cellular exercise, it isn't really necessary to present yourself in the accepted exercise positions. Cowboys,.Indians and the Cavalry go plenty of rebound exercise while sitting astride a steed. There are those, however who do not have a choice. For some reason, they are not able to stand. That doesn't have to prevent them from participating in aerobic. strength, and health exercises. Amputees and wheel chair pilots alike can enjoy the quality of exercise they desperately need by rebounding in a sitting position.

And don't sell the sitting position short. Some of the greatest athletes use the sitting position to strengthen their abdominal and trunk muscles. Try sitting in the middle of your unit, lean back, lift your legs so that you are sitting in a V position, and then establish your bounce by rhythmically moving your arms forward and up. The equal and opposite reaction will force your body into the mat.

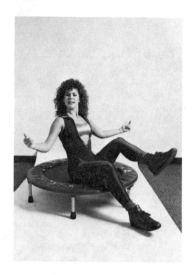

By reversing the movement of your arms at just the right time, you will be able to develop a bounce. Don't be discouraged if you are not able to do this one at first. This is one of the harder, more demanding rebound movements. I can only think of one harder and that is doing the V bounce. That one is done by adding the bicycle movement of the legs while bouncing in the V position.

All of the above are single movements which can be performed over and over again without much thought or the need for concentration. But they can also be interwoven into a routine, with or without music. A smooth transition from one movement to another and still another and, "Look Ma, I'm dancing!"

A well-choreographed rebound dance routine becomes a work of art. What was just a form of exercise then transcends its original purpose. Instead of merely working the body, an esthetic flow of movement fascinating to watch, and to perform, is achieved. And isn't that the normal evolution of all man's achievements?

Gymnastics and body-building started out in the dark and smelly basements of old buildings. Now, they are performed in the sophisticated homes of connoisseurs of body movement.

Buildings were originally built as simple shelters. Now they are meant to say something about the builder, the owner, the city, and the rest of the surrounding environment. As others discover rebounding, it too will evolve. Already, there have been attempts at rebound competition in Texas and Florida. And they won't be the last.

CHAPTER 8

PHILIPPINES
MY FIRST MEDICAL AUDIENCE

Near the end of April, 1983, I received an invitation from President and Mrs. Marcos of the Philippines to go and do the same thing there that had been accomplished in Hong Kong. My flight arragements back to the States included a one-week visit to the "country of a thousand islands." I was more that a little surprised when my airplane was met by a military escort. As soon as I was identified as I got off the plane, one of the guards stepped forward and placed a nut lei around my neck. I was told to move to the center of the formation, and with four military men in front and four behind me marching two abreast, we marched smartly right through customs to a waiting limousine. Although we didn't dally along the way, my luggage was already in the trunk by the time we arrived curbside. I am easily impressed. They didn't have to do it, but it was an experience I'll never forget. Two motorcycles and a secret service automobile in front of the limo and the same behind I felt was a little too much. But that was the way

I was taken to my luxury hotel in Manilla. The flowers and fruit basket in my room were only a token of how I was to be pampered during my stay.

The next day, I was given a tour of the University built by Mrs. Marcos and donated to the youth of her country. In the presence of her personal physician, my visit with Mrs. Marcos lasted an hour and a half. "What's your opinion?" Mrs. Marcos asked her doctor.

"This is something I believe all medical doctors need to hear," was his surprising reply.

"That's just what I was thinking," she replied. "Will you make the arrangements?"

"Yes, Ma'am. Mr. Carter, would Thursday afternoon at one o'clock be alright with you?"

"I am at your service." I said. That was Tuesday. I spent all day Wednesday preparing for the meeting by going to their medical library and reserving their copy of *Medical Physiology* by Arther C. Guyton, M.D., Morris' *Human Anatomy*, edited by J. Parsons Shaeffer, and several other books in their library I hadn't seen before. If I had any chance at all to impress the doctors, I was going to have to meet them on their turf with their books.

Philippines - My First Medical Audience

I was at the hospital before noon on Thursday checking out the lecture hall. It had a well-lit stage two feet high and ten feet deep across the front of the room. I requested, and immediately got, a wireless lapel mike that was tuned in to the state-of-the art in-house public address system. The room was set up for two hundred people. I was hoping for twenty-five. At 12:45, the first of the what was to be an audience of seventy-five nurses and fifty medical doctors began to arrive and take their seats. I selected three nurses and invited them to sit at a table next to the stage. I placed the books I had selected the day before in front of them and gave them instructions to look up and read what I asked them to read when I asked them to read it.

The closer it got to 1:00, the more I began to realize the importance of this meeting. This was the acid test of the many theories of rebound exercise. If I was going to be shot down, this audience would be able to do it. Was I ready to handle the humiliation if they got up and walked out? What if I couldn't answer their questions to their satisfaction? Do they believe in lynching foreign "quacks?" Maybe I should walk out. I wondered how far it was to the airport. At 1:05, the doors closed. Too late. They made my introduction too flowery. Where did they get all that information about me anyway? Through the buzzing in my head I heard,

". . . in for a unique experience. Please welcome, Dr. Albert Carter."

I'm no doctor, I thought, as I shifted mental gears from my personal pessimism to my public optimism. I reached to the back of my belt and turned on my wireless mike as I moved center-stage. I remember my presentation to that elite audience as if it happened yesterday.

"Thank you. I see you've done your homework, however, I'm not a doctor. I am a trampolinist and an author. I write about trampolining. I am here in front of you because something I said to Mrs. Marcos was valuable enough to her to cause her to request this meeting.

"Today, we are going to talk about the health benefits of exercise. I am not going to talk about your need for exercise, because I'm sure you already know how important exercise is to the overall health of the human body. In the next few minutes, I am going to introduce to you a form of exercise that, until recently, has been completely overlooked. It's an activity that has been around for over fifty years in the United States but has never been considered by our experts as an exercise. This activity is known as rebound exercise, the same type of exercise you would receive if you had access to a trampoline.

"A basic understanding of how all exercise affects the body will help you understand rebound exercise. . ." I remember establishing the fact that the common denominator of all exercise is the opposition to the gravitational pull of the earth. This caught their attention, because they had never thought of exercise in this light. Exercise has always been used to stimulate muscles. When I pointed out that the forces of acceleration, and deceleration were facts of life but that we had not taken advantage of them when it came to exercise, they became emotionally involved with the discussion.

"The vertical stacking of these three forces by rebounding has got to be one of the greatest breakthroughs in health maintenance!" I remember surprising even myself by making that statement. I backed it up by explaining that rebounding is a cellular exercise, that we were no longer concerned about stimulating only the muscle fibers to greater strength, but that every cell in the body had the ability to adjust to external stimulations. This included bone, nerve, and connective tissue cells. There is no reason to believe that this cellular stimulation does not include even the vital organs and hormone-producing organs of the endocrine system.

They applauded the aerobic exercises, and were amazed at the simplicity of the strength exercises. But I believe I made the greatest impact when I began to talk about the lymphatic system.

"You all know where the blood pump is. The heart starts beating before you are born and continues to beat until you die. But it only pumps blood. It does not pump lymph fluid. You have three times as much lymph fluid in your body as you do blood. Lymph fluid surrounds the tissue cells of the body. When the cells of the body need nutrients, they have to get it from the lymph fluid. When they excrete metabolic waste, it goes into the lymph. Obviously the more circulation your lymph fluid receives, the healthier you are going to be.

The problem is that we have never taken this mystifying system seriously. For example, we are able to hear the heart, measure the beat, monitor the pressure of the blood. But, because the lymphatic system just quietly goes about its job, not making waves, we don't study it. In fact, we have done just the opposite. Because we don't understand its importance, we have tried to get rid of it. We started forty years ago by removing the tonsils and the adenoids from healthy children, two of the drainage organs of the lymphatic system. We have no love for the appendix, another lymphatic drainage organ. Removal is in order every time a surgeon gets close to one. Lymph veins are stripped from the arms during a mastectomy. Until recently, the lymphatic system was just a big bother to the surgeon.

"A description of the lymphatic system will help you understand how rebounding actually multiples the day-to-day function of this extremely important system." I turned to the three nurses sitting at the table and asked, "Would you please turn to page 361, in *Medical Physiology,* and read the very first paragraph of Chapter 31, the chapter on the lymphatic system?"

A lovely musical voice came over the in-house public address system.

"The lymphatic system represents an accessory route by which fluids can flow from the interstitial spaces into the blood. And, most important of all, the lymphatics can carry proteins and large particulate matter away from the tissue spaces, neither of which can be removed by absorption directly into the blood capillary. We shall see that this removal of proteins from the interstitial spaces is an absolutely essential function, without which we would die within about 24 hours."

"Tell me, does that paragraph indicate that lymphatic circulation is important?"

I received nods of agreement and a few murmured "yesses" from the audience. Then I let them have it.

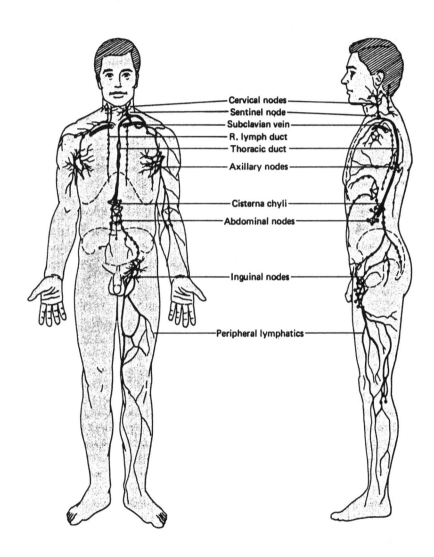

Cervical nodes
Sentinel node
Subclavian vein
R. lymph duct
Thoracic duct
Axillary nodes

Cisterna chyli
Abdominal nodes

Inguinal nodes

Peripheral lymphatics

The Lymphatic System

"Since the lymphatic system is not connected up to the heart, how does the lymph circulate? I would like to have all of you hold up your right hand. (I could not believe I was doing this with doctors and nurses, but they played along and each held up a right hand.) Now, hold up your first finger on that hand." (They did.) "With that finger please point to your own personal lymph pump." I paused and waited. The fingers stayed pointed in the air and the audience began to murmur, indicating to themselves and to me they didn't have any idea whether they had a lymph pump, let alone where it was.

I turned to the three nurses sitting at the table at the foot of the stage, "Would you please turn to page 363 in *Medical Physiology* and read the big bold print at the bottom of the second column?"

The book was opened and another lovely voice read over the speakers,

"The Lymphatic Pump."

"We all have a lymphatic pump." I stated emphatically. The question now is how can we turn it on?" I turned again to the table and asked, "Would you please turn the page and read the second paragraph beginning with, 'obviously'?"

The same voice read,

"Obviously, the lymphatic pump becomes very active during exercise, often increasing lymph flow as much as 10 to 30 fold. On the other hand, during periods of rest lymph flow is very sluggish."

"Now, why is it that exercise has such a great effect on the lymphatic pump, and what exercise has the greatest impact?" I asked my audience. "Both answers can be found in the description of the pump." I exclaimed, answering my own question. "Would you please read the paragraph beginning with 'The Lymphatic Pump'?"

"Valves exist in all lymph channels, even down to the tips of the lymphatic capillaries. In the large lymphatics, valves exist every few millimeters, and in the smaller lymphatics the valves are much closer together than this."

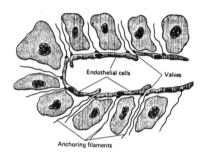

"In other words, the lymphatics is a hydraulic pressure system made up of tubes or veins which start at the lymphatic terminals, or minute internal vacuum nozzles. The walls of the veins at the nozzles are only one-cell thick. But as they combine, the veins become thicker and stronger. They drain into the lymph nodes where the lymph fluid is filtered and foreign invaders are destroyed. Other larger veins drain the lymph nodes into even larger veins. They finally empty into the thoracic duct, which is as thick as your thumb. All of the veins are filled with millions of one-way valves. Any time there is pressure below the valves, they open. Greater pressure above the valves will keep them closed. The up-and-down motion while rebounding activates the one-way valves to their maximum. And it happens approximately a hundred times a minute. In fact, if all of us had little red labels across our forehead, that said, 'Shake well before using', we would all be healthier!" They laughed. The doctors actually laughed.

When I opened up the lecture for questions and answers, every time a question was asked from the floor, I turned to my table of nurses and books and asked them to read the answer to the audience.

Question: "Mr. Carter, How do you know that exercise, and

more specifically rebounding, has any effect on the immune system?"

Answer: "Thank you. To answer that, we need to know the relationship between the lymphatic system and the immune system. Please turn to page 60 and read the first two sentences."

"The human body has the ability to resist almost all types of organisms or toxins that tend to damage the tissues and organs. This capacity is called immunity. Much of the immunity is caused by a special immune system that forms antibodies, and activated lymphocytes that attack and destroy the specific organisms and toxins. This type of immunity is acquired-immunity. However, an additional portion of the immunity results from general processes. This is called innate-immunity."

"Thank you. Now, continue with the third paragraph of the second column of the same page."

"We shall see that both the antibodies and the activated lymphocytes are formed in the lymphoid tissues of the body."

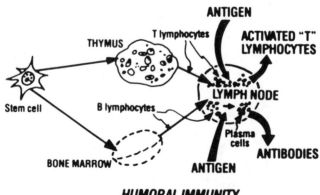

CELL-MEDIATED IMMUNITY

ANTIGEN

T lymphocytes

THYMUS

ACTIVATED "T" LYMPHOCYTES

Stem cell

B lymphocytes

LYMPH NODE

Plasma cells

ANTIBODIES

BONE MARROW

ANTIGEN

HUMORAL IMMUNITY

"To find out where the lymphoid tissue is found, read the first line of the fourth paragraph of page 61."

"The lymphoid tissue is located most extensively in the lymph nodes."

Question: "Mr. Carter, I thought that the T-lymphocytes were manufactured in the Thymus and the B-lymphocytes were manufactured in the bursa, or bone marrow. Can you explain the apparent discrepancy?"

"Actually, both types of lymphocytes are derived originally in the embryo from pluripotent hemopoietic stem cells. After which, they receive further education, or preprocessing from the thymus or bursa, but to answer where they go afterwards, turn to page 62, fourth paragraph."

"After formation of processed lymphocytes in both the thymus and the bursa, these first circulate freely in the blood for a few hours, but then become entrapped in the lymphoid tissue."

"So, you see, the activated lymphocytes, whether manufactured by the T-lymphocytes and the antibodies, or manufactured by the B-lymphocytes are sent out into the rest of the body from the lymph nodes. The speed with which they

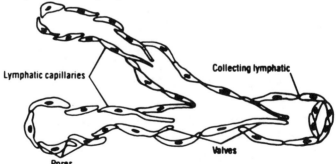

are dispatched is dependent on the speed of the lymph-flow through the lymph nodes. If I could increase this function by 10 to 20 fold by exercising, I would surely make sure I would do it daily."

Question: "Are you trying to tell us that rebounding makes many medicines obsolete?

Answer: "Not I. I am not a doctor, so I do not have the authority to say such things. Let's turn to the book all medical doctors have accepted as authoritive and see what it says. First, we need to understand the immune system's first and second lines of defense. Please read the second column on page 56 beginning with *The Tissue Macrophages.*"

"The macrophages that are already present in the tissues immediately begin their phagocytic action. Therefore, they are the first line of defense against infection during the first hour or so. However, their numbers are not very great."

"I'm sure you will agree with me that the macrophages are the same cells as the monocytes. The only difference is that the monocytes are immature cells freshly formed in the bone marrow and found in the bloodstream. As soon as they leave the bloodstream through the small holes in the capillary walls, they swell to five times their original size and become macrophages capable of destroying hundreds of bacteria by eating them."

"Now, read the following paragraph."

"Neutrophilia means an increase in the number of neutrophils in the blood. Within a few hours after the onset of acute inflammation, the number of neutrophils in the blood sometimes increases as much as four- to fivefold - to as high as 15,000 to 25,000 per cubic millimeter."

"Thank you. Recall, if you will, that the neutrophils are only one-fifth the size and capability of the macrophages, but usually out number them about ten to one." Please turn to page 57, and read the second paragraph."

The book was passed down to the third nurse. She read:

"Almost any factor that causes some degree of tissue destruction will cause neutrophilia. For instance, persons debilitated by cancer exhibit an increase in neutrophils from the normal of 4500 per cubic millimeter sometimes up to 15,000 or more."

"That's good." I said. "Now read the fourth paragraph of the same column."

"The number of neutrophils in the circulatory system can increase as much as two to three times normal after a single minute of extremely hard exercise. . ."

"Good. And the next paragraph."

"Approximately one hour after physiological neutrophilia has resulted from exercise, the number of neutrophils in the blood is usually back to normal."

"Do the neutrophils remain in the bloodstream?" I asked the audience.

"No." a doctor volunteered.

"Please explain." I requested.

"All lymphocytes have the ability to leave the blood stream by *diapedesis,* or squeezing through holes smaller than they are, and travel to the source of infection by *chemotaxis.*"

"Once they leave the bloodstream, where are they?" I asked.

"In the lymph fluid surrounding the cells." I heard from several of the nurses.

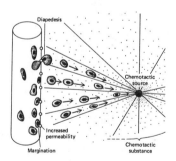

Question: "The concept of cellular exercise is intriguing because we have only thought of exercising groups of muscles. Do you have any reason to believe that the individual lymphocytes actually become stronger, thereby making it faster and easier for the lymphocytes to get to the scene of the infection or injury?"

Answer: "That is a very good question. I have two references. First, let's see what gives the muscle the ability to contract. Please turn to Chapter Eleven, page 120, *The Contraction of the Skeletal Muscle,* and read the first paragraph."

"Approximately 40 percent of the body is skeletal muscle and almost another 10 percent is smooth and cardiac muscle. Many of the same principles of contraction apply to all these different types of muscle."

"Thank you. To find out what the principles of contraction they are talking about, let's go to page 121, third paragraph."

"Each muscle fiber contains several hundred to several thousand myofibrils, which in turn has lying side-by-side, about 1500 myosin filaments and 3000 actin filaments, which are large polymerized protein molecules that are responsible for muscle contraction."

"Are we agreed, then, that the ability of the muscle to contract is dependent upon the interaction of the actin and myocin molecules?"

There was a general agreement from the audience.

"And we do agree that exercise does strengthen muscles." Again, a general nodding.

"Then, please turn with me to page 24, first paragraph and lets find out how lymphocytes move."

"It is believed that ameboid locomotion is caused in the following way: The outer portion of the cytoplasm is in a gel state and is called the ectoplasm, whereas the central portion of the cytoplasm is in a solid state and is called endoplasm. In the gel are numerous microfiliments composed of actin, and also present are many myocin molecules that interact with the actin to cause contraction the same as occurs in muscle."

Question: "Mr. Carter. Do you have the whole book memorized?"

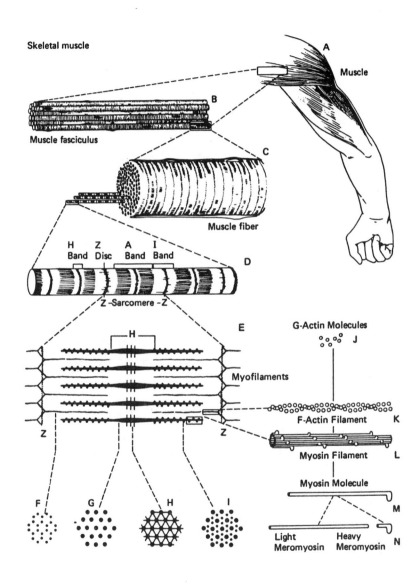

Skeletal Muscle

Answer: "Just the important parts. I've had to defend my position on cellular exercise for so long that it became necessary to be prepared.

"Now, if cellular exercise is a valid concept, then scientists will come up with the same conclusion. Let me refer you to a study published in the *Physiologist Magazine,* December 1979." Again, I turned to the table and asked, "What is the title of the study you have in front of you?"

"Human Lymphocyte Activation is Depressed at Low-G and Enhanced at High'G."

"How many doctors involved with the study?"

"Seven."

"Where did it take place?"

"Zurich."

"What lymphocytes were involved?"

"They were taken from the cosmonauts and astronauts."

"How active were lymphocytes after space flight, or low G?"

"About 50% of the control group at 1 G."

"After spinning them around in a centrifuge creating a 1.8 G environment for three days, how active were they compared to the control?"

"At least twice as active."

"In fact, it says, 'Analysis of the ultrastructure by electron microscopy shows that at high G cells are more swollen and richer in vacuols than at 1G.' So you see, it is entirely possible that cellular exercise does exist, and that rebounding creates the necessary high G environment necessary to increase the strength and activity of the individual lymphocyte, thereby increasing the efficiency of the entire immune system."

A Gratifying Conclusion

The meeting lasted a total of two and a half hours. At the end, I was mobbed by those who wanted more information. to call it a success seems too tame, yet I know of no other way to describe the results.

"That was the greatest demonstration of subject comprehension I have ever seen!" exclaimed the Head Surgeon as he came up to thank me for my demonstration.

"Thank you. Coming from you, that is the greatest compliment I have ever received." I returned, seriously.

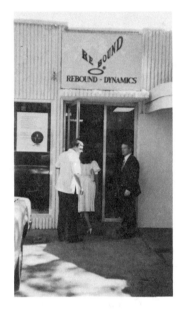

We established a Rebound Dynamics office in the Philippines and even demonstrated rebounding on the streets of Manila to enthusiastic audiences.

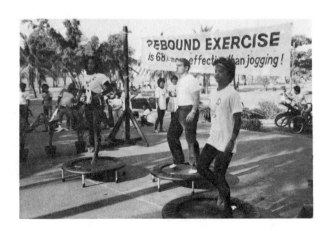

CHAPTER 9

NASA
CLIMBS ON MY BANDWAGON

My sense of accomplishment and worth to my fellow man made me feel as if I could almost fly home to Seattle without the assistance of United Airlines. My faith was not sufficient, so I used my airline ticket. Four months after leaving my family for a ten-day lecture visit to Australia, I landed back into the waiting arms of a loving and very patient family. Among the hugs and kisses and stories of unshared experiences, came the news, "You have a letter from NASA on your desk at home!" Darren blurted, not able to keep his excitement contained any longer.

"What's that all about?" I asked Bonnie, knowing that she wouldn't have an answer.

"I don't know. It came just a couple of days ago."

"Why would they be writing to me?"

" 'Cause you're famous," piped Melynda.

"I hope it doesn't mean another trip," smiled Bonnie.

"Probably not," I said, all the time thinking, "Why not? Rebound exercise is just as important to the people here in

124

the United States as it is to those in Hong Kong or the Philippines."

The NASA Communique

National Aeronautics and
Space Administration
Washington, D.C.
20546

06 May 1983

Mr. Albert Carter
125 Nineth Ave. North
Edmonds, WA 98020

Dear Mr. Carter:
Dick Orrick has told me of the interesting conversation he had with you regarding rebound exercise, and we hope the effect of NASA research in rebounding will prove sufficient to meet publication tests for Spinoff 1984.

As Dick mentioned, we are careful to avoid making false claims in the Spinoff articles. It is therefore hoped that you can justifiably attribute to NASA some contribution to the acceptance or development of rebounding as a medically safe and efficient body exercise.

The material you are to furnish, including cassettes, will be useful background information for our purposes. In your cover letter please describe how you believe the NASA research impacted rebounding.

It appears that rebounding could be the subject of an interesting article in Spinoff 1984, and we look forward to receiving your materials. Attached for your perusal is a copy of Spinoff 1982.

Sincerely,

Leonard A. Ault
Chief, Dissemination &
Analysis Office
Enclosure

I guess to most people, this would be a compliment. To me, it was a slap in the face. Not just a little slap from an insignificant human being, but a major, bowling over, crippling blow from the elite scientific arm of the greatest country in the world!

It seemed to me that they wanted to take credit for the discovery of rebound exercise, now that it was successful in other countires. They wanted to put a story in their official publication showing the rest of the world how their scientific investigation provided the foundation of rebounding. If it were not for the investigation, publication, and advertising of The National Institute of Reboundology and Health, Inc., nobody would even know that NASA was the least bit interested in rebound exercise. Their study comparing trampolining to jogging would be still locked up in the catacombs of the libraries around the world gathering dust.

I pulled myself up short. Now, wait a minute, Al. The information you have accumulated about rebound exercise has been because many people contributed bits and pieces along the way. How can you use this invitation to increase the potential of sharing rebounding with others? I will first call and find out how much NASA knows about rebound exercise, how much they are using it, and volunteer to help them understand it even more. Good idea. I have their letter, a name, and a phone number. That's all I need to secure an invitation to at least talk - maybe an audience who knows?

The first call was to Washington D.C., where I was referred to a phone number in Houston, where I was referred to a name in California, closer to home. 'I have them coming my way.' I mused.

"Yes, this is Ames Research Center on Moffett Field. . . There are so many scientific studies going on here that it would be impossible to tell if that study was done here . . . If it was published in the *Journal of Applied Physiology* stating that it was done here, then it must have been done here. . . I'll ring that department for you."

"Yes, I do remember that study, Mr. Carter, but all of the scientists who participated have since been transferred or have taken positions with other corporations. Therefore, it would be impossible to continue that study because of the start-up costs involved to bring together another study group. . . Yes, I am aware that comparitive results were astounding. . . 68% more efficient than jogging? Well, If we published it, we were fairly sure of our results before it was published. . . Of course, that is reason to continue to study, Mr. Carter. But before we study anything, we have to secure the budget, the personnel, and the facilities. Even before that, there has to be a request for the study from somebody with authority. That hasn't happened, and I don't see it happening anytime in the future. However, if you happen to be in the area, please stop in. What you say sounds interesting. I could bring together a few doctors to hear your presentation."

That was all I needed. I now had an invitation to talk to the NASA scientists. I would make sure I "just happened" to be in that area within the next two weeks.

Presenting Rebounding to NASA

Six doctors. That was actually better than I expected on such short notice. They were all Ph.Ds in Exercise Physiology and other health-related fields. They were responsible for the health of the astronauts before, during, and after space flight. The two hour discussion went as I expected - skeptical at first - warming near the middle - and super enthused at the wrap up.

Conclusion #1. Astronauts could use rebound exercise before space flight to get in shape because it is a cellular exercise utilizing the very forces they will be experiencing during space flight.

Conclusion # 2. Astronauts need rebound exercise after space flight to overcome the atrophy caused by zerogravity. In a flight lasting only fourteen days, they lost up to 15% of bone and muscle mass. Hard surface jogging would be devastating on astronauts suffering from space-induced osteoporosis. The G force loading would reverse the G force unloading in space.

Conclusion #3. We need to consider the positive effects of the forces of acceleration and deceleration to take the place of gravity in space. We are developing an exercise method called 'Off-the-Wall' exercises. An astronaut in free-flight will push off the wall, turn a half sommersault, and land on an opposite wall, thereby creating a 1 G effect each time direction is changed.

CHAPTER 10

HOW TO MEASURE YOUR IMPROVEMENT

I am constantly asked to compare the effects of rebound exercise to that of other exercise activities, such as walking or jogging. The accepted means of comparison in the exercise world is the aerobics method presented to us by Dr. Kenneth Cooper, in his series of books on Aerobics. His method was simple if all you wanted to do was measure the amount of calories burned. That is sort of like measuring an automobile by the quantity and quality of exhaust coming from the tailpipe. Although this will give you an accurate measurement of fuel consumption, it will not tell you the quality of the internal environment of the automobile, or the body. We live in a world of measurement and calibration. We want somebody to tell us how much is "good" and how much is "too much" almost to the point where we are willing to listen to people who know nothing about the body.

The best method of exercise evaluation is simple. Listen to your body. When you know how, it will tell you when you have had enough or when you need more.

Here are three rules of thumb you can use as you exercise by rebounding:

1. Because of the many and various benefits you will get out of rebounding, we have found that five times a day is better than three, and three is better than one. Please be careful of any exercise program or method where the experts tell you to exercise three times a week. The reasoning behind that 48 hour lay-off is because that exercise method is too hard on the body and the body needs time to heal. Rebounding is not traumatic. You can exercise many times each day without any ill effects.

2. If you are interested in developing endurance, rebound until you are huffing and puffing, then continue as long as it is comfortable. Keep in mind, there is nothing magic about 20 minutes, 12 minutes, or any other length of time. If you are breathing hard, you are improving your endurance.

3. Never go through a pain threshold. You have an internal doctor telling you when you have had enough. The idea that you have to be in pain and must strain to gain and train is for the ignorant coaches who haven't heard of a better way.

As soon as you understand and use these simple rules, nobody will have to tell you how much exercise you need again. It is about this time that I receive the question from somebody, "Shouldn't you see a doctor if you are over forty-five before you start rebounding?" The answer to that is simply, "If it will make you feel better." In other words, if you have any reason to believe that exercising could be life-threating to you, by all means, see your doctor. But don't procrastinate beginning rebounding because you haven't had your physical examination. I have prepared some exercise programs to help you design one for you. These programs are here just to give you an idea of what others are doing. If you do not find one that fits you, develop one of your own. After all, there is only one you.

ACTIVITIES EVALUATION CHART

5 Points = Poor   10 Points = Good   15 Points = Excellent

Activity	Calories Used Per Hour 114 lb.	154 lb.	194 lb.	Muscular Development	General Endurance	Flexibility	Balance	Safety	Convenience	Frequency	Frequency Points	Total Points
Rebound-sprint	1260	1440	1710	10	15	15	15	15	15	3 day	105	430
Jumping rope	590	750	930	5	10	5	15	5	15	1 day	35	215
Running	590	750	930	10	15	5	10	5	15	3 wk	15	200
Skiing	630	810	990	10	10	10	15	5	5	occ	5	195
Swimming-butterfly	780	840	900	15	15	15	10	10	5	1 wk	5	215
Rebound-strength	870	1050	1230	15	15	15	15	15	15	5 day	175	440
Basketball	510	630	750	10	10	15	15	5	10	3 wk	15	185
Bicycling-15 mph	510	890	810	10	15	5	10	10	15	1 day	35	210
Swimming-back stroke	480	600	600	15	15	15	10	10	5	1 wk	5	175
Weight lifting	540	660	780	15	5	5	5	10	10	3 wk	15	170
Football	480	600	720	10	10	10	10	5	5	1 wk	5	155
Karate	420	540	660	10	5	10	10	5	5	3 wk	15	150
Mountain climbing	480	600	720	15	15	10	10	10	15	occ	5	165
Rebound-jogging	480	600	720	10	15	15	15	15	15	5 day	175	365
Bicycling-10 mph	360	420	480	10	15	5	5	10	15	1 day	35	170
Calisthenics	300	360	420	10	5	10	5	15	15	1 day	35	155
Dancing	270	330	390	5	10	5	10	10	15	1 wk	5	120
Table tennis	270	330	390	5	5	10	10	10	15	1 day	35	140
Walking-outside	300	360	420	10	10	5	15	15	15	1 day	35	150
Rebound-health	90	150	210	5	10	15	15	15	15	5 day	175	280
Walking-indoor	90	150	210	5	10	5	5	15	15	5 day	175	255

SUGGESTED EXERCISE PROGRAM

	6 a.m. (½ hr. before breakfast)	11:30 a.m. (½ hr. before lunch)	5:30 p.m. (½ hr. before dinner)	Daily Min. Totals
1st wk.	1 min. health 1 min. aerobic	1 min. health 2 min. aerobic	1 min. health 2 min. strength	
5 days/wk.	2 min. total	3 min. total	3 min. total	8 min./day 40 min./wk.
2nd wk.	2 min. strength 2 min. health	1 min. health 3 min. aerobic	1 min. health 3 min. strength	
5 days/wk.	4 min. total	4 min. total	4 min. total	12 min./day 60 min./wk.
3rd wk.	1 min. health 2 min. aerobic 2 min. strength 1 min. health	1 min. health 3 min. aerobic 1 min. health	1 min. health 4 min. strength 1 min. health	
5 days/wk.	6 min. total	5 min. total	6 min. total	17 min./day 85 min./wk.
4th wk.	2 min. health 3 min. aerobic 3 min. strength 1 min. health	2 min. health 4 min. aerobic 1 min. health	2 min. health 4 min. strength 4 min. aerobic 1 min. health	
5 days/wk.	9 min. total	7 min. total	11 min. total	27 min./day 135 min./wk.
5th wk.	2 min. health 5 min. aerobic 4 min. strength 1 min. health	2 min. health 4 min. aerobic 3 min. strength 1 min. health	2 min. health 5 min. aerobic 4 min. strength 1 min. health	
5 days/wk.	12 min. total	10 min. total	12 min. total	34 total/day 170 min./wk.

Suggested Rebound Exercise Programs

Rebounding is now being used by men and women and boys and girls from all walks of life for numerous reasons. Some people want to gain weight, others want to lose weight. Executives want to control stress, while the youth want to develop a better sense of balance while building muscle, bulk and strength. Some of the women are preparing for a "blessed event", while some have been too blessed. Whatever your reason, with a little bit of imagination, you will never have a reason for saying that rebounding is boring, unless, of course, you are just bored with your life.

Adults: Weight control and body tone are of primary concern, muscle strength and balance are secondary. Nevertheless, feeling good and looking good are the reasons most adults exercise.

ADULTS

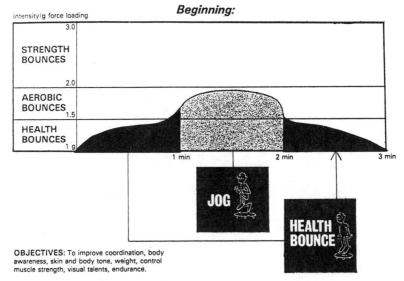

OBJECTIVES: To improve coordination, body awareness, skin and body tone, weight, control muscle strength, visual talents, endurance.

ADULTS

Intermediate:

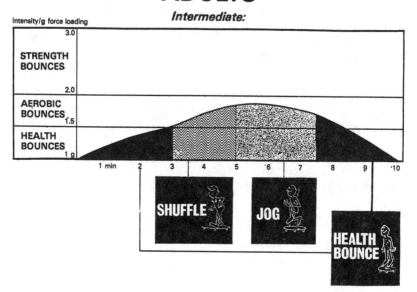

ADULTS

Goal:

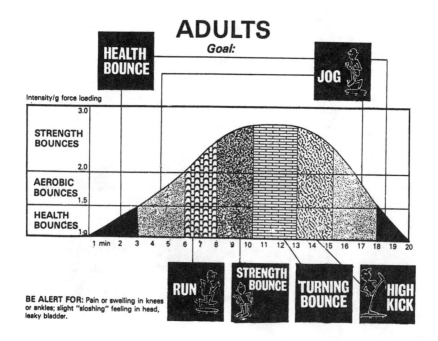

BE ALERT FOR: Pain or swelling in knees or ankles; slight "sloshing" feeling in head, leaky bladder.

Executives: The objective is balance and coordination, stomach muscle and back strength, mental alertness, stress control, weight control, memory improvement, and, for some, an improved golf score. Time efficiency is a major concern for executives when they exercise.

Most exercise programs require at least two hours from the time the individual changes clothes, drives to a facility, warms up, exercises, showers, changes clothes, and drives home. Time is money. Our objective is to show the executive that he or she can eliminate coffee breaks, and replace them with rebound breaks. Rebounding is a positive requirement for good health. You can get a full exercise program everyday without using up any of the company's precious time.

If possible, have the rebound unit in the office next to your desk, or in a meeting room. By the way, a ProBounder 2000 can be in the boardroom during those long meetings when you tend to fall asleep. All you have to do is get up and rebound and you will be alert again and not miss any of your meeting. It beats nodding off in your chair.

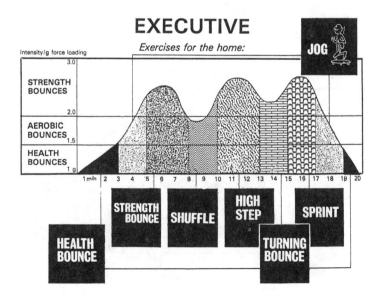

EXECUTIVE

Exercises for the office:

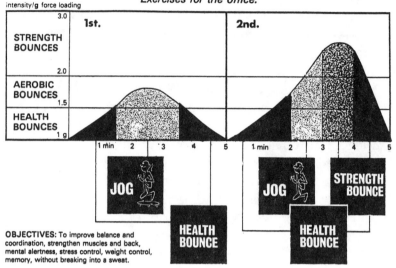

OBJECTIVES: To improve balance and coordination, strengthen muscles and back, mental alertness, stress control, weight control, memory, without breaking into a sweat.

EXECUTIVE

Exercises for the office (cont.):

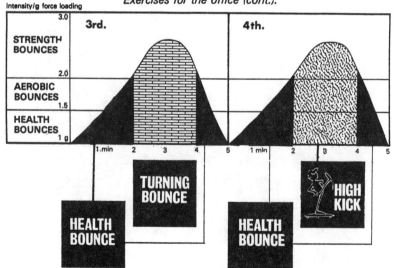

Senior Citizens: The objective for the senior citizen is balance and coordination, muscle and bone strength, endurance and health. Put the ProBounder 2000 next to the wall for support.

Exercise should consist mainly of the health bounces, the aerobic bounces, and very mild strength bounces. Therapeutic redounding identifies the weakest part of the body and exercises only that part, constantly strengthening it while stimulating the rest of the body. As soon as these weak spots are properly strengthened, you can exercise the rest of the body by simply becoming more vigorous. Remember, it is not necessary to ever go through a pain threshold.

SENIOR CITIZENS

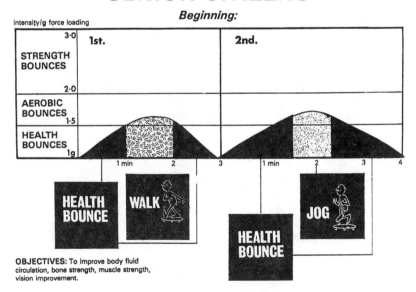

Beginning:

OBJECTIVES: To improve body fluid circulation, bone strength, muscle strength, vision improvement.

SENIOR CITIZENS

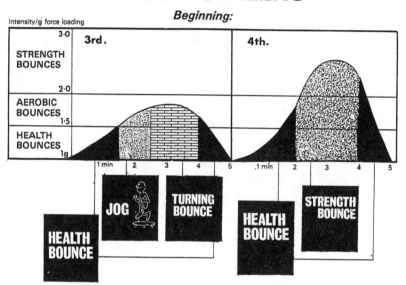

SENIOR CITIZENS

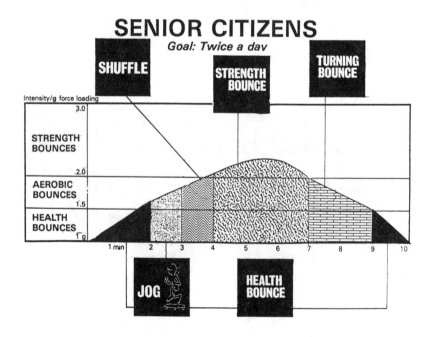

Pregnancy: When a woman finds she is pregnant, she has less than nine months to prepare for the greatest demand on her body - childbirth. The better shape she is in, the easier and safer it will be for both mother and child. Generally, exercise is good. Most medical authorities agree that exercise is proper for the pregnant woman, especially a mild cellular exercise.

However, exercise should be limited to a mild health bounce and a mild aerobic bounce. In the aerobic bounces the legs are moving up and down vigorously and the body is fairly stationary - it is the mat that gives. If you have any reason to think you will have complications, check with your doctor before you begin.

PREGNANCY

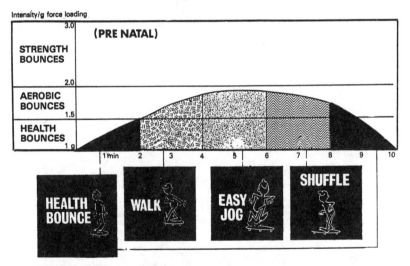

OBJECTIVES: To improve body circulation of mother and child, muscle strength, bone strength.

After Childbirth: In the early seventies, shortly after jogging became an accepted way of life for many, gynecologists began to receive more visits from women complaining of abdominal discomfort. These women were told that they had prolapsed organs, meaning that the ovaries, uterus or bladder had torn away from the proper position and fallen to the bottom of the abdominal cavity. This was prevalent among women afer child birth because many attempted to get back their pre-pregnancy figure by keeping pace with their husbands' aerobic workout.

All the vital organs are held in place by connective (anchor) tissues, made up of cells. These become weaker with disuse, and stronger under rebounding resistance.

After childbirth, it's necessary for the mother to start easy exercises to tone and tighten her body. Most doctors recommend sit ups, which develop the abdominal muscles, but nothing for skin tissue. Rebounding not only exercises the abdominal muscles, but also tones and tightens the skin tissue, cell by cell. Childbirth also tends to leach bones of calcium and other important minerals, leaving them weak. Rebounding stimulates bones to become stronger, mineralized, and dense.

PREGNANCY

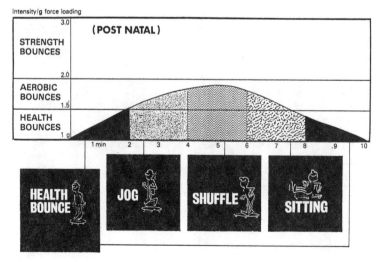

Youth: Just as you are concerned with your child's nutritional health and provide him or her with multiple vitamins, you should consider a multiple exercise program. Regardless of your child's activities, you can be assured of the proper stimulation of the neuro-muscular system necessary for motor skills.

This is not to be a strict regimen, but one to show what is needed by the young as their bodies grow. There will be times when they will be clumsy, stumbling over themselves. The author of *How to Improve Your Child's Intelligence* Dr. G. N. Getman, says that everyone should be involved with trampolining. In other words, the clumsier the child, the more he or she should be involved.

The young bones of the skeletal system grow rapidly, sometimes growing so fast that the joints and bones become weak. The effect of rebound exercise on the weight-bearing joints and the bones concerned with compressional stress provides an environment which demands greater strength.

Your child is never too young to start rebounding.

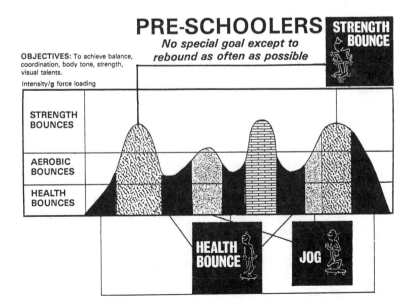

YOUTH

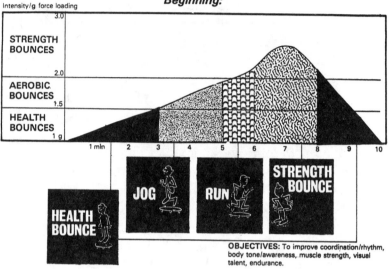

Beginning:

OBJECTIVES: To improve coordination/rhythm, body tone/awareness, muscle strength, visual talent, endurance.

YOUTH

Goal:

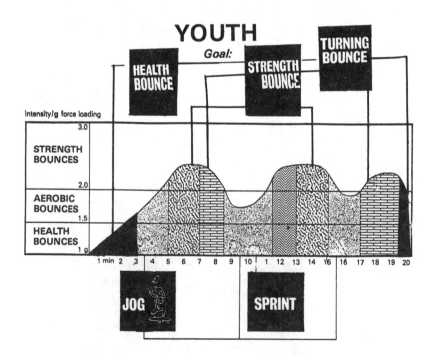

Summary

You will notice that we merely mention the vision improvement techniques of rebound exercise, rebound education, theraputic rebounding, and rebound exercise and the athlete. And although we have included enough information to help you get started in your own personal exercise program at home, or in your office, please don't think we have covered all that could be said about the health benefits of rebound exercise. We have only just begun. I have left out much, simply because, to do each subject justice, each deserves a book of its own. Keep in touch. We'll let you know when they are available. Some are in rough manuscript form now waiting to be polished.

CHAPTER 11

THE HEALTHY CELL CONCEPT

As universally necessary as rebounding is to each and every cell in the body, I would still be remiss indeed if I failed to touch on the other three requirements of each of the body's 75 trillion cells. I originated *The Healthy Cell Concept* back in 1982. I've been preaching and teaching it ever since, usually in the closing minutes of a Reboundology Seminar.

Although others have picked up on this concept (some even go so far as to claim erroneously to have originated it), the first book to contain the true Healthy Cell Concept is *The Cancer Answer*. The co-authors of *The Cancer Answer* are Albert E. Carter (in my persona as Professor Carter, a university instructor of physiology), and Larry Lymphocyte (a highly-schooled white blood cell), one of the top guns of the immune system. This miniature molecule has more tricks of the trade at his disposal than a legendary Green Beret. With thorough and very authoritative documentation, Larry pokes holes in

144

accepted medical and scientific theory regarding cancer. In spite of Professor Carter's able defense of the establishment position, Larry proves that cancer myths are preventing our scientists from eradicating cancer. But that's another story.

As the author of *The Cancer Answer*, modesty prevents me from suggesting that you rush out and buy this very entertaining and highly-informative book. However, *honesty* compels me to tell you that you'll almost certainly learn more about how to prevent (and conquer) cancer (and any other condition of ill health) by reading this book than you could possibly glean from any other single source. True words. But enough about that book. This chapter is about The Healthy Cell concept.

The Basic Needs of The Healthy Cell

Each of us begins life as a single cell. A cell transforms itself into two identical cells by a process known as *mitosis,* or cell division. Each daughter cell carries the identical DNA programming with which the organism was endowed at the instant of conception. This incredible process of multiplication by division continues until at last the adult human is made up of a mass of 75 trillion highly-intelligent and very knowledgeable cells. Each individual cell knows its business and performs its function in concert with all others.

Each of our 75 trillion cells requires tender loving care. As long as we adequately tend to the care and feeding of the community of cells which comprise our bodies, we live and prosper in health. This fact is so basic to life itself that no authority will argue against it. The Healthy Cell Concept precisely identifies the basic needs of the cell. Simply living the simple precepts of The Healthy Cell concept gives you a very real edge in the health and longevity sweepstakes.

Divided into four equally important parts, the following chart shows you exactly what your cells, and therefore *you,* require for abundant health.

Larry Lymphocyte co-author of *The Cancer Answer*

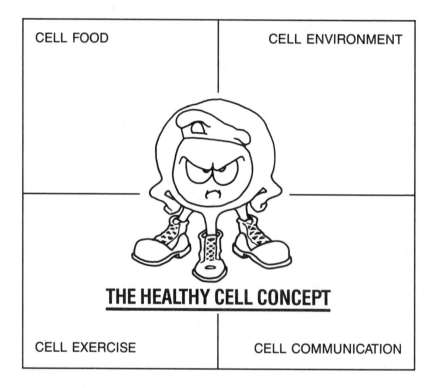

CELL FOOD	CELL ENVIRONMENT
CELL EXERCISE	CELL COMMUNICATION

THE HEALTHY CELL CONCEPT

Cell Food

If your cells had the ability to do the marketing, you would find only whole unprocessed foods in their shopping cart. The reason for this is very simple. All the chemicals and preservatives and dyes and artifical flavorings and processing agents and so on ad infinitum that have found their way into the food chain are alien elements which your immune system has to defend against.

When the white blood cells of the immune system are scurrying around cleaning your body of all these foreign invaders, they scarcely have time to do the important work they were originally assigned by the Creator of us all. The cells of the immune system (primarily leukocytes, lymphocytes, neutrophils, macrophages) need to be about their serious task of searching out and ridding the body of mutant cells (precancerous, cancerous), invading viruses, dead, diseased or infected cells, and metabolic trash. Think about it.

The solution is obvious, isn't it? Provide your body with the nutrients your cells need; avoid the alien elements the immune system has to defend against.

One of the best complete cell foods available to us is bee pollen. Pollen is the very essence of the living plant and contains the blueprint of the plant itself. The obliging bees flit from flower to flower selecting only the most powerfully nutritive golden dust within their flying range. By the time they return to the hive with laden pollen baskets, the dusty golden pollen has been transformed by their industry into tightly-packed bee pollen granules about the size of a Grape Nut. And each golden granule is a powerhouse of nutrition literally bursting with vitamins, minerals, amino acids, hormones, enzymes, carbohydrates, and trace elements.

Besides being a complete food, another quality your cells will really appreciate is the fact that bee pollen is a live food. All that delicious nutrition is 'manufactured' by mother nature. It pleases me to report that science has not been able to synthesize this perfect live food in a laboratory. Why? Bee pollen contains some mysterious *extra* factor that so far defies analysis. Some authorities believe that it's this little bit of magic added by the bees that makes bee pollen such a highly beneficial cell food.

How else to explain the fact that, according to Dr. William Robinson of the USDA, bee pollen added to food exerts an anticarcinogenic effect? In his 1948 study, Dr. Robinson reported that in mice bred to develop mammary tumors, most of those given bee pollen failed to develop a tumor at all and existing tumors shrank. The control group not given bee pollen with their feed wasn't so lucky. All developed cancerous tumors and died right on schedule.

Quality is very important when you're shopping for bee pollen. If it's incorrectly harvested, stored, or processed, it can very easily lose a lot of its goodness. You might not be able to tell the difference between brands, but, believe me, your cells can. I favor the raw Desert Gold Bee pollen granules from Bio-San. I find this multiblended bee pollen delicious 'as is' and spoon it right out of the bag. For those who prefer capsules, the Desert Gold people offer Bee Pollesan. This capsule formula contains top quality Desert Gold Bee pollen, plus royal jelly and two herbal potentiators, ginseng and gotu kola.

While we're on the subject, there's some excellent bee pollen 'candy bars' on the market, too. The CC Pollen company started it all with their President's Lunch, a delicious bar containing bee pollen, honey, oats, sunflower seeds, peanut butter, and other good-tasting naturals. The President's Choice is the same bar swathed in carob. This company also puts out several other bars. They're all low in calories and richly nutritive, making any of them an excellent choice as a meal replacement in a weight-loss program, as well as a healthy snack.

Two other products of the beehive, propolis and royal jelly, deserve a mention here, although they might be more properly termed 'Cell Ammunition,' than cell food. For instance, propolis is the strongest natural antibiotic around. Science confirms that propolis has antiviral, antibacterial, and antifungal properties as well. In regular use, propolis helps ward off coughs, colds, and flu. Sometimes called the 'longevity factor,' royal jelly is another excellent product produced naturally by the bees. Royal jelly aids cell rejuvenation, stimulates hormonal production, and assists the glandular systems of the body.

Another very important cell food that I supply my cells with every day is cold-pressed unrefined C-Leinosan Linseed Oil. Unlike most U.S. produced vegetable oils, even the ones legally labeled cold-processed and unrefined, this product is truly a raw unrefined product with all the essential fatty acids and enzymes intact. The experts have determined that the body must be supplied daily with linoleic and linolenic fatty acids, termed essential because the cells cannot manufacture these fatty acids from any other nutrients. Unfortunately, the typical American diet is lacking in the essentials.

I always take my C-Leinosan with low-fat cottage cheese because Germany's premiere biochemist, Dr. Johanna Budwig, has clinically proven that the sulphurated amino acids in cottage cheese paired with the essential fatty acids in unrefined linseed oil combine dynamically in the body to produce highly beneficial effects.

This seems to be the place to clear up the confusion surrounding the terms *linseed* and *flax*. According to any source you consult, including the *Encyclopedia Britannica*, the two are identical. Botanically speaking, both linseed and flax are used interchangeably to identify the plant *Linum usitatissimum.* The *Britannica* also tells us that Linum usitatissimum is cultivated both for the fiber in the stem, called *flax,* from which linen yarn and fabric are made, and for its seed, called *linseed,* from which linseed oil is obtained. Because it is impossible to produce linseed oil (or flax oil) by processing the stem of the plant, the term 'flax seed' oil is actually a misnomer, although it is commonly and popularly used interchangeably with the correct term, which is linseed oil.

When chemically extracted, or extracted by the usual screw-press which generates extremely high temperatures (although this oil can be legally labeled unrefined and cold-pressed in the U.S. because no *external* heat is applied), any oil thus produced is lacking in the essential fatty acids and contains chemically-alien metabolites. Although unrefined linseed oil is used both as a good food and as a therapeutic with very impessive credentials abroad, U.S.-produced linseed oil is most often used as a drying agent in the manufacture of paints and varnishes and so on. The linseed meal leftover after the oil is extracted is pressed into cakes and used as a food for livestock, but it's tainted with chemicals and the nutrient content is greatly reduced because of the heat which has been generated by the friction of the press.

You also should know that the world scientific community universally selects unrefined linseed oil as their unanimous choice when researching the benefits of the essential fatty acids. I have read reams of such research. When correctly cold-pressed, crude, and unrefined, linseed oil is the richest source of the essential fatty acids known to man *and* the important live enzymes are not destroyed. And that's why I favor C-Leinosan Linseed Oil.

Another company producing good cell food in supplement form is *Fountain of Health.* As long as a supplement is produced in strict accordance with an all-natural formula and isn't mucked up with colors and dyes and chemical preservatives and artificial gunk, your cells can't tell the difference between a correctly-produced supplement and the good whole foods you ought to be putting on your dinner plate. In other words, if your menu is lacking in the important nutrients which science has determined preserve and protect life and health, you can take a good supplement to fill the gaps.

For instance, garlic has been used by healers since the days of antiquity. This smelly herb has antiseptic, antibacterial, antifungal, and bacteriostatic properties. In regular use, garlic assists the immune system, helps normalize the metabolic rate, increases energy levels, and is a body cleanser of heroic proportions. But few of us are such fans of nature's own preventive 'medicine' that we care to include a clove or two of garlic in our daily diet. In capsule form, *Garlic Plus* provides all the benefits of this legendary botanical medicinal. Plus, this one is naturally deodorized with parsley, synergistically potentiated with cayenne, and contains no unwanted additives.

Another important dietary factor is the fiber you find in whole grains and fresh vegetables. The American Cancer Society, the American Heart Association, and the AMA all tout the benfits of fiber. If you're eating on the run, or are still using quick-fix processed convenience foods, you might consider *Fiber Plus.* This supplement supplies organic fiber from seven major fiber groups, plus the important minerals (calcium, magnesium, zinc) which the body loses quickly when the optimum amount of fiber is present in the diet. Supplying your body with the fiber it needs has been shown to overcome chronic constipation, helps establish good bowel habits, aids digestion, and cleanses the entire gastrointestinal tract.

Rebounding itself promotes strong bones and is a documented osteoporosis preventive. But, if dairy products aren't present in sufficient quantity in your diet, *Calcium Plus* can take up the slack. This important formula supplies organic calcium, phosphorus, and magnesium in an easily-assimilated form.

Are carrots a favorite in your household? If not, think *Beta-Carotene Plus.* These caps are produced from especially-grown Dunaliella Kona originating in sunny Hawaii. Dunaliella Kona is an abundant source of natural beta-carotene, and is far richer in this protective nutrient than carrots themselves. As the precursor of vitamin A, beta-carotene is an important element which the body uses to produce vitamin A as needed. Another plus, all-nautral Beta-Carotene Plus is stabilized with the natural antioxidants, vitamins C and E.

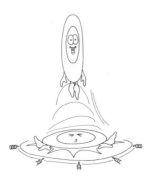

Cell Exercise - Because this entire book is devoted to explaining 'The Miracles of Rebound Exercise,' I hardly need to expand on the topic here. For the incredible number of benefits inherent in rebound exercise, suffice it to say that rebounding is a very important part of The Healthy Cell Concept. Only rebounding perfectly fits the parameters of the perfect Cell exercise.

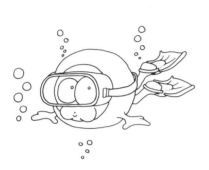

Cell Environment The internal environment of your body is the home of your more than 75 trillion cells. By weight, 57 percent of your body is water. About 25 percent of this water is termed intracellular fluid, protoplasm, or cytoplasm and is *inside* your cells. The other 32 percent is known as extracellular fluid or interstitial fluid and is *outside* your cells. This is the internal environment where the cells live and function.

Your cells depend on the constant mix of your body fluids for their supply of water, oxygen, hormones, and nutrients. Most people are surprised to learn that there's three times as much extracellular fluid in the body as there is of blood. Water is more important to your cells than any other of the categorized nutrients, including vitamins, minerals, proteins, carbohydrates, or fats. In fact, water is more important to life than all nutrients combined. Cells need water for every cellular activity. Water is critical to efficient kidney function and waste removal. Water is required to control your body temperature. It is also an absolutely essential solvent and the transport system for many nutrients, including some important vitamins you can't live without. Water lubricates your digestive tract and cushions your joints. It is an essential part of the protective system of your eyes, both inside and out. Blood is almost all water, and, another surprise, bones are more than 20 percent water. Water is the universal solvent. It can get through all of your cell membranes in order to take nutrients in, or waste material and hormones out.

Unfortunately, drinking the water that comes into your home and flows out of your tap is almost certainly hazardous to your health. For example, most community water systems supply heavily chlorinated water which they call 'purified' and which is considered to be of acceptable potable, or drinking quality. And a great many community water systems also routinely add flouride as a decay preventive to the drinking water they deliver to local homes. Let's look at these two chemicals one at a time.

Chlorine is a nonmetallic element, a diatomic gas that is heavy, noncombustible, and greenish-yellow. It is toxic and irritating to skin and lungs. Besides purifying water, chlorine is used in the manufacture of carbon tetrachloride and trichlorethylene and in shrink-proofing wool. It's put in flame retardant compounds, and used in processing fish, vegetables, and fruit, primarily because chlorine kills bacteria and other things that would otherwise cause fresh foods to rot.

True, chlorine does destroy the waterborne bacteria which causes typhoid fever, cholera, and dysentery. But chlorine injures red blood cells and damages their ability to carry life-giving oxygen where it's needed. Chlorinated water cannot be used for kidney dialysis. And the chlorine used to kill bacteria in drinking water may contain carbon tetrachloride, a contaminant formed during the production process. Chlorinating water has also been shown to cause the formation of other undesirable chemical compounds in water, such as toluene, xylene, and styrene. To the cells of your body, these chemicals are deadly. They kill off red and white blood cells, destroy skin cells, and produce serious heart problems. Chlorine and other harmful chemicals are present in virtually every water supply tested.

Research shows there's a 44 percent higher incidence of gastro-intestinal and urinary tract cancers in populations drinking chlorinated water than in matching control groups drinking non-chlorinated water. Over 10 years ago, U.S.S.R. scientists discovered that people drinking water containing 1.4

milligrams ppm (parts per million) of chlorine had higher blood pressure readings on average than those drinking water with only .3 to .4 milligrams ppm of chlorine.

Fluoride, a waste byproduct of aluminum manufacture, should properly be termed *fluorine* because it's one of the halogen group of chemicals. The other three are chlorine, bromine, and iodine. If a human were to ingest 1 milligram of sodium fluoride, approximately 45 percent of it would be fluorine, and the rest would be sodium. Fluorine is an insidious poison. It's toxic, very harmful, and cumulative in effect. Even when ingested in minimal amounts, fluorine remains in the tissues and builds up over time. No matter how many sources call it 'safe,' the fact remains that fluorine is one of the poisons our cells must defend against.

The Grand Rapids-Muskegon study is often cited in support of artificially fluoridating city water. However, five years into what was supposed to be a ten-year study, fluoride advocates found that the decay rate of non-fluoridated Muskegon was decreasing at the same rate as fluoridated Grand Rapids. Because this data didn't support fluoride, Muskegon was dropped from the study as the control city. The published report states only that tooth decay dropped in Grand Rapids, inferring that fluoride caused the decrease. Thanks to some spectacular publicity, the general population was easily convinced that fluoridation is a good thing. But studies by the U.S. Public Health Service show no difference in tooth decay rates between high and low fluoridated areas. British, Danish, and Japanese studies all agree that fluoride does not reduce the incidence of tooth decay.

Remember, it is a documented fact that as little as one-tenth of an ounce of fluoride can cause death. When sold over-the-counter, fluoride comes in a can marked with the universal symbol of poison, the skull and cross bones. The optimal amount of fluoride is advertised to be 1 part-per-million. But the ingestion of drinking water containing as little as 1.2 to 3 ppm of fluorine will cause such developmental disturbances in bones as osteosclerosis, spondilitis, and osteoporosis, and goiters as well. Scientists at the Siebersdorf Research Center in Austria have reported that as little as 1 ppm of fluoride slows down the activity of the immune system and can cause various genetic and chromosomal damage in plants, animals, and humans. Using bone marrow and testes cells, a U.S. geneticist has demonstrated that the degree of chromosomal damage increases proportionally in direct relation to the amount of fluoride in water.

Using the same level of fluoride commonly put into U.S. drinking water. Scientists at the Nippon Dental College of Japan have determined that even this minute amount of fluoride is capable of transforming normal cells into cancer cells. At a meeting of the Japanese Association of Cancer Research in Osaka in 1982, the researchers reported: "Last year at this meeting, we showed that sodium fluoride, which is being used for the prevention of dental carries, induces chromosomal abberrations in the irregular synthesis of DNA. This year, we report findings that show malignant transformation of cells is induced by sodium fluoride."

It's easy to see that, when your internal Cell Environment is contaminated with poisons your immune system has to try to defend you against, the cells of the immune system become overworked and exhausted. Without the full participation of your immune system cells, you get sick - or worse. On top of the need to search out all the cells in your entire body which have been damaged beyond repair by the poisons in your water, the immune system cells must also try to neutralize and rid the body of all the waterborne contaminates you drink every day. Scary, isn't it?

I've named two of the very common chemicals, chlorine and fluoride, which are almost certainly present in your drinking water. I'm not even going to bring up the agricultural and manufacturing agents and other pollutants that are seeping into our groundwater supplies. I'm not going to talk about the carcinogens and particulate matter and viruses and worse which have been identified in the drinking water in far too many areas.

It would appear that no source of pure drinking water still remains anywhere on the planet. Yet, water is necessary to sustain life. The solution is obvious: a water purification system which removes the bad and leaves the good. Reverse osmosis is the one water purifying system which does just that. Although city officials will point out that using reverse osmosis to cleanse drinking water for an entire city is too costly, I could counter with: "How much is too much for a life-sustaining element?" But, until the cost of this process becomes much lower, if then, city water supplies will probably continue to be heavily chlorinated in the name of 'purification' and fluoridated in the name of 'tooth decay prevention.'

Be that as it may, a supply of pure drinking water is a necessity. A word of caution is in order here. Water bottled in plastic, even if prepared by reverse osmosis, may contain harmful hydrocarbons which have leached out of the plastic container. This water certainly tastes better than the chemicalized stuff that flows from your tap, but it's still not the best choice.

The answer, of course, is a home purification system which operates on the reverse osmosis principle. Simply put, reverse osmosis forces water to flow through a semipermeable membrane. (This same principle is used to cleanse the blood in kidney dialysis.) Pure water, H_2O, is composed of hydrogen and oxygen. The semipermeable membrane allows the tiny hydrogen and oxygen molecules to slip through easily, but the larger molecules which make up chemical agents (including chlorine and fluoride), particulates, viruses, and all kinds of harmful dissolved solids, are too big to pass through the special membrane and are flushed down the drain into the sewer where they belong.

It was the U.S. Government who researched and developed

the reverse osmosis water purification process at great expense. Purifying water by reverse osmosis is deceptively simple, but very, very effective. Polluted tap water containing who knows how many dangerous combinations of chemical elements, is forced through a semipermeable membrane, using only the water pressure behind the flow. No electricity or energy source is required to operate the process, making it very, very economical. Once the system is in place, you'll be generating safe pure water at around one cent per gallon. The drawing below shows how it works.

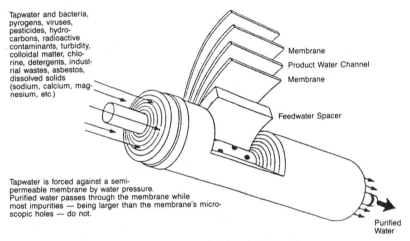

Tapwater and bacteria, pyrogens, viruses, pesticides, hydrocarbons, radioactive contaminants, turbidity, colloidal matter, chlorine, detergents, industrial wastes, asbestos, dissolved solids (sodium, calcium, magnesium, etc.)

Membrane

Product Water Channel

Membrane

Feedwater Spacer

Tapwater is forced against a semipermeable membrane by water pressure. Purified water passes through the membrane while most impurities — being larger than the membrane's microscopic holes — do not.

Purified Water

Reverse Osmosis Filter/Membrane

Many of the pollutants in our water are tasteless, odorless, colorless, and dissolve (and disappear) in water. On top of the chemicals which give your water a bad taste and chemical smell, there's a lot you can't identify, but they're there nonetheless. The list includes viruses, bacteria, parasites, inorganic salts, dissolved metals, asbestos fibers, pesticides, herbicides, radioactive particles, trihalomethanes and other poisonous chemicals, such as fluoride, chlorines and chloramines. Every year hundreds of new chemical compounds are created, greatly compounding the existing problem.

Once you have a reverse osmosis system hooked up to your kitchen faucet, you can relax. All the harmful pollutants are filtered out and flushed down the drain. The water that emerges from your tap is crystal-clear pure and sparkling water with a neutral taste composed of 2 parts hydrogen and 1 part oxygen, as nature intended.

There is just no way to overemphasize the importance of securing a pure source of drinking and cooking water. All those pollutants make a lot of extra *unnecessary* work for your immune system cells. When your white blood cells (lymphocytes, leukocytes, macrophages, neutrophils) have to take the time to clean up the dangerous contaminants you've ingested along with your drinking water, they can't be about their *real* business of searching out and destroying mutant cells, carcinogenic (cancer) cells, viruses, infected cells, harmful bacteria and on and on.

After investigating a great many water purification systems, we decided on the *Fountain of Health Purwater Reverse Osmosis Water Purifiers*. These units remove bacteria, viruses, pesticides, agricultural and industrial chemicals, soaps, dissolved solids (including asbestos fibers) - chlorine and fluoride - everything *but* the H_2O molecules. This company backs up their results with hard scientific data, something many water purifier manufacturers can't do. The chart (see right) documents the *Purwater* results.

We are well satisfied that the Purwater people do it right. Especially important is the fact that you can select from a variety of Purwater systems sized - and priced - to fit any household. From the small portable model, just right for traveling or a small household, to the reasonably-priced counter-top unit, to the convenient permanently installed under sink model, there's one that's just right for you.

No matter which Purwater unit you select, we just cannot overemphasize the importance of using *only* pure water. Your

The Purwater Reverse Osmosis Water Purifying System

KEY: ○ YES ● NO ◐ SOME

POLLUTANT	ENERGY SOURCE	Purwater Reverse Osmosis (WATER PRESSURE)	De-Ionization (RESIN—ION EXCHANGE)	Distillation (ELECTRIC-CONDENSATION)	Activated Carbon Filter (WATER PRESSURE)	Sediment Filter (WATER PRESSURE)
UNPLEASANT TASTE/ODOR		○	●	●	○	●
SEDIMENT		○	●	○	◐	○
PESTICIDES		○	●	○	○	●
CHLORINE		○	●	◐	○	●
RADIOACTIVE CONTAMINANTS		○	●	◐	●	●
DIOXIN		○	●	○	●	●
Trihalomethanes (THM) Trichloroethylene (TCE)		○	●	◐	●	●
ORGANICS		○	●	◐	●	●
ALKALINITY		○	◐	◐	●	●
FLUORIDES		○	○	○	●	●
CHLORIDES		○	○	○	●	●
PHOSPHATES		○	○	○	●	●
MAGNESIUM (HARDNESS)		○	○	○	●	●
CALCIUM (HARDNESS)		○	○	○	●	●
SULFATES		○	○	○	●	●
POTASSIUM		○	○	○	●	●
CADMIUM		○	○	○	●	●
LEAD		○	○	○	●	●
ARSENIC		○	○	○	●	●
SODIUM		○	○	○	●	●

PURIFICATION: Purwater Reverse Osmosis · De-Ionization · Distillation

FILTRATION: Activated Carbon Filter · Sediment Filter

ı SILVER ACTIVATED CARBON

initial expense is offset by the fact that you'll be spending only a penny per gallon for safe, pure water for all your needs. If you use a credit card.

Although these reverse osmosis water purifiers are not inexpensive, the benefits in terms of your health are incalculable. Truly, the quality of your life and health depends on the quality of the water you put into your body. That's medically and scientifically documented *fact*. The government isn't doing it for us, you know. It's up to you to make sure that the water your body depends on to maintain and sustain life isn't undermining it instead. Make sure it's pure.

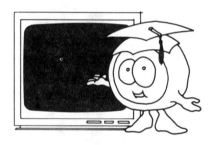

Cell Communication - Have you ever wrestled unsuccessfully with a problem just before you went to sleep only to find the appropriate action occurring to you when you awaken in the morning? Whatever you input just before you fall asleep becomes of vital concern to your brain cells. While you're sleeping, your mind is actively working. Many times, if you have a problem you find difficult to solve, just concentrate on it before you go to sleep. You'll awaken to find the solution ready and waiting.

You communicate with your cells constantly. They communicate both among themselves and with you constantly. Through a series of intricate neurotransmitters, your cells register pain instantaneously when you inadvertently burn yourself in the kitchen. You snatch your hand away from a hot handle without thinking. And you don't have to think before scratching an itch. Almost before you realize you've got one, your fingers are automatically scratching away.

Every time you learn something, anything at all, it is indelibly recorded in the DNA of all the cells charged with the responsibility of retrieving some information or reconstructing an action when called upon. Whether it is the cells of your brain recalling a memory or the cells of your muscles and the nerves of your fingertips as you type, or the big muscles of your legs as you run and jump, your cells learn as you learn.

At times, we are guilty of sending our cells a message that can be harmful to our health. When that happens, your cells become confused about things they instinctively know are right for you. It becomes a dangerous situation when your cells are not acting in your best interests because you're sending out the wrong singals.

Let me give you a 'worst case' scenario. Suppose someone you care deeply about is diagnosed as having cancer and is told by his doctor he has just six months to live. His immune system cells detected the cancer long before he or the doctor were aware of this threat to the health of the body and were already hard at work battling the malignancy. The diagnosis of cancer, or any other possibly terminal condition, puts a person under a great deal of stress. When a patient is given a death sentence by his doctor, this message runs through the body like a shot of adrenalin. When the cells of the body perceive the individual has given up, they simply prepare the body for death. The cells also give up and quit fighting. The immune system slows down and becomes inefficient, giving the cancer an opportunity to take over.

You communicate with the cells of your body by your attitude. More important than any almost any other single factor to your total cell environment is your attitude toward life. A positive winning attitude puts all the cells of your body on notice that perfection is expected in the functioning of your body. There are documented cases of individuals who have overcome all odds and performed seeming miracles because they refused to accept physical illness.

Medical scientists call that 'psycho-immunity' and it involves strong visualization. A cancer patient might imagine that his immune system cells are white knights in shining armor and his cancer is a dragon. He continually sends his white knights out to fight the dragon and eventually the knights triumph. True, your cells automatically battle the 'cancer dragon.' But, when a patient is thinking positive thoughts, he isn't poisoning his internal environment with negative messages. Visualizing a hard-fought internal battle and winning out is very favorable to your cells. This message is communicated throughout the body. All cells feel they are part of a winning team and remember that what they do really matters. All the cells of the body will pull together with perfect confidence that all the other cells will do their part. And so they will.

The phsycial laws of the body are irrevocably decreed and recorded in the DNA upon which your health is predicated. When you receive the blessings of good health, it is by obedience to those laws upon which health is predicated. Your good health is not accidental. It takes a lot of hard work on the part of your cells to keep your healthy, and you must do your part.

Cellular communication can come in the form of prayer, hopes, dreams, visualization, and even direct verbal commands. We might take the old saying: "As a man thinketh in his heart, so he is," and carry it one step further: "As a man thinketh in his cells, so he is." Your cells are so intimately aware of the way you regard yourself that many of the illnesses man experiences we bring on ourselves.

Worry, fear, anger, anxiety, and guilt are examples of feelings that we all experience from time to time. When we allow these negative thoughts to persist, our hormone-producing glands send destructive messages to the cells. The cells listen, obey, and react almost instantaneously. Some cells begin to produce chemical messages of doom and destruction, which are transmitted to other cells of the body. These messages are misinterpreted by the rest of the cells. In turn, they respond by misfunctioning. A chemical imbalance can show up as hives, allergies, rashes, or twitches. Sometimes we call it 'stress' and let it go at that. At other times, symptoms of a chemical imbalance can mimic an illness, and are classified and treated as such.

Correct cellular communication is vitally important. The power of positive thinking is very real. Take care that the messages you transmit to your cells by your every thought and action are feelings of robust health and vitality. And know that your cells will hear and obey.

CHAPTER 12

CLOSING COMMENTS

A lot of you have been waiting a long time for this updated revised second edition of *The Miracles of Rebound Exercise*. During the intervening 10 years, I've made what I believe is good use of my time. I have a lot more solidly documented information to pass on to you this time than I did back in the early years of rebounding. Of course, *I* always knew that rebounding is the most effective and most efficient form of exercise ever devised by man, it's just that *now* it's been scientifically proven. After reading this book, I hope you'll agree that it's been worth the wait.

And, to you 'orphans' among those reading this book, the vast number of people who bought a rebound exercise device from a store that couldn't provide you with the information you needed to make use of the device, probably because they didn't understand the powerful tool they sold you themselves, welcome home. If you have a decent rebounder that's been gathering dust in the back of the garage because you didn't really understand what to do with it, now you know. Start bouncing!

If you don't have a ProBounder 2000, but you're ready, willing, and eager to get started experiencing the benefits of this form of exercise, the superior quality, long lasting ProBounder 2000 is easy to find. Top sporting goods stores and some health-good stores carry them. Most of the fine natural products I discussed in The Healthy Cell Concept are available in better health-food stores, too. Call your favorite local store and ask. If you prefer the convenience of armchair shopping, New Dimensions Distributors services the entire nation through their efficient mail-order department. If you'd like one of their catalogs, here's how to get in touch:

New Dimensions Distributors
16548 E. Laser Drive
Fountain Hills, Arizona 85268
Call 1-800-624-7114 Toll-Free Nationwide
In Arizona (602) Call: 1-837-8322

I'd like to remind you of one last thing before I write 'The End' and wrap up this book. No one is too young to start rebounding. No one is too old to begin rebounding. No one is too frail for rebounding. No one is too physically disabled for rebounding, even though some may need a little help from a friend. Rebounding can be tailored to the condition and goals of the user. Everyone from an Olympic athlete in training (who needs a challenging routine) to an aging and ailing senior (who responds positively to the gentlest bounce) will benefit from rebounding. In short, rebounding is the one ideal universal exercise, the one true cellular exercise, the most effective and efficient form of exercise ever devised.

What are you waiting for? Ready, set, BOUNCE!

CHAPTER 13

N.A.S.A. CONFIRMS IT!

Rebound exercise is "The most efficient, effective form of exercise yet devised by man."

". . . for similar levels of heart rate and oxygen consumption, the magnitude of the biomechanical stimuli is greater with jumping on a trampoline than with running, a finding that might help identify acceleration parameters needed for the design of remedial procedures to avert deconditioning in persons exposed to weightlessness."

The above statement is one of several made in a scientific study published in the Journal of Applied Physiology 49(5): 881-887, 1980, which confirms many of the statements previously made in the "Miracles of Rebound Exercise". The research was performed by the Biomechanical Research Division, NASA-Ames Research Center, Moffett Field, California, in cooperation with the Wenner-Gren Research Laboratory, University of Kentucky, Lexington, Kentucky.

The four scientists, A. Bhattacharya, E.P. McCutcheon, E. Shvartz, and J.E. Greenleaf, secured the assistance of eight

166

young men between the ages of 19 and 26 to each walk, jog, and run on a treadmill which was operated at four different speeds and then jump on a standard sized trampoline at four different heights to compare the difference between the two modes of exercise. Although treadmill running had been studied many times before, the scientists found that "... *measurements of the necessary variables have not been reported previously for trampoline exercise.*" The trampoline testing was conducted at least one week after the treadmill testing.

The six measurements which were taken on all eight of the subjects were:

1. A pulse before exercising.
2. A pulse immediately after exercising.
3. The amount of oxygen consumed while exercising.
4. The amount of G-force experienced at the ankle while exercising.
5. The amount of G-force experienced at the lower-back while exercising.
6. The amount of G-force experienced at the forehead while exercising.

The pulse was obtained by a battery-powered electro-cardiographic unit taped to the subject's body which transmitted its signals to a custom-designed receiver which in turn recorded the information by electronically writing it on a chart.

The oxygen consumption was measured with a K-meter which the subject carried on his back.

The G-force experienced by the ankle, back and forehead of each of the university students was measured by small sensitive accelerometers which were placed in plexiglass holders that were taped to the ankle, the small of the back, and the forehead.

After a thorough medical examination, the healthy students were issued a pair of shorts and new Nike running shoes to standardize the conditions to be measured. They were given familiarization sessions on laboratory procedures, treadmill running and trampoline jumping to ensure the exercise techniques would be the same. Each student then walked or ran four different speeds on the treadmill with a five to ten minute rest period between runs while the scientist recorded their statistics and compared them with previous treadmill studies for accuracy.

A week later, these same athletes returned to bounce on a trampoline at four different heights with a 5 to 10 minute rest period in between exercise sessions. Again the scientists recorded their statistics, only this time, they had no previous studies to compare them to. Since trampolining had not been previously studied, the only studies available were the preliminary studies which began in August of 1977 on passive restrained humans and animals exposed to increasing frequency and amplitude of vibration forces designed to increase heart rate and metabolic activity. *"These responses measured by whole-body vibration resemble those during mild exercise and suggest that perhaps body vibration could be used in place of exercise."*

The results of this study were startling to the scientists but quite frankly, were expected by us at the "Institute". Following are some of the results revealed by this team of scientists from NASA:

1. The G-force measured at the ankle was always more than twice the G-force measured at the back and forehead while running on a treadmill.

This helps to explain shinsplints and knee problems, especially when the natural shock absorbing system of the body becomes so fatigued that it doesn't do its job correctly, thus throwing added unexpected forces on already tired muscles, ligaments and tendons, forcing them beyond the point of rupture.

2. While jumping on a trampoline, the G-force was almost the same at all three points, (ankle, back,

forehead) and well below the rupture threshold of a normal healthy individual.

This makes it possible to exercise the entire body knowing that there is no undue pressure applied to part of the body such as the feet, ankles, and legs, and at the same time knowing that each part of the body is receiving the necessary environmental stresses it needs to become stronger cell by cell.

3. The external work output at equivalent levels of oxygen uptake were significantly greater while trampolining than running. The greatest difference was about 68%.

The efficient use of the vertical forces of acceleration and deceleration to produce internal loading by directly opposing the gravitational pull develops more biomechanical work with less energy expended, thus less oxygen used and less demand placed on the heart.

4. While trampolining, as long as the G-force remained below 4-G's, the ratio of oxygen consumption compared to biomechanical conditioning was sometimes more than twice as efficient as treadmill running.

It is important to note that although this experiment was performed on a trampoline where the participants were able to develop a G-force as high as 8-G's, the efficient use of energy was below 4-G's. People involved in rebound exercise on rebound units have been measured only as high as 3.5-G's, so that any activity on a rebound unit is more efficient than treadmill running at any speed.

5. With the G-force the same as or greater than 4-G's *". . . there was no significant difference in the oxygen uptake between the two regimens".*

Even when a person is able to develop a force on the trampoline of more than 4-G's, although it is no more efficient as far as oxygen consumption than running, it is still much better on the lower extremities because the cells are still below their rupture threshold providing a safe way to exercise.

6. *". . . averting the deconditioning that occurs during the immobilization of bed rest or space flight, due to a lack of gravireceptor stimulation (in addition to other factors), requires an acceleration profile that can be delivered at a relatively low metabolic cost. . . for equivalent metabolic cost, and acceleration profile from jumping will provide greater stimuli to gravireceptors."*

This statement verifies the fact that rebound exercise is an excellent exercise for our senior citizens, those physically handicapped, those who are recuperating from an accident or injury, or anyone else who needs exercise but is hampered by a pre-existing physical condition.